Fasting Keto Diet

Create an Unstoppable Fat-Burning Force by Uniting Ketosis with Intermittent Fasting

Thomas Rohmer

Disclaimer:

This guide has been created for informational and reference purposes only. The author, publisher, and any other affiliated parties cannot be held in any way accountable for any personal injuries or damage allegedly resulting from the information contained herein, or from any misuse of such guidance. Although strict measures have been taken to provide accurate information, the parties involved with the creation and publication of this guide take no responsibility for any issues that many arise from alleged discrepancies contained herein. It is strongly recommended that you consult a physician, personal trainer, and nutritionist prior to commencing this or any other workout or diet plan. This guide is not a substitute for professional personal guidance from a qualified medical professional. If you feel pain or discomfort at any point during exercises contained herein, cease the activity immediately and seek medical guidance.

Table of Contents

Introduction:

Weight loss is without a doubt a difficult thing to pull off. Every year millions of people unsuccessfully try to lose weight and end up failing. You might've tried to lose weight in the past and failed as well.

Was it your lack of determination? Did you not give it all you had? Or maybe it was your diet plan that set you up to fail before you even started.

Sadly, most diet plans out there focus on quick results and short-term changes. Sure, gimmicky diets can help you lose 20 pounds in a month, but then you get thrown to the wolves once the diet ends. What are you supposed to be able to do to keep the weight off for the rest of your life? Unfortunately, that's your problem to figure out and not the diet's.

The company that sold you the diet plan or supplement doesn't care about your results. In fact, they want to see you fail so that you'll come back and buy the next latest and greatest thing that's (supposedly) guaranteed to work! If you were actually successful with keeping the weight off, then what else would there be left to sell you?

Luckily, you're in the right place. I'm not here to sell you on any overhyped powder or potion, and I care about you getting lasting results that you'll be proud of. I'm going to share with you one of the most powerful (and sustainable) approaches you can take to lose weight. Many people know about intermittent fasting and the ketogenic diet. However, people rarely think to combine the two diets in order to create an unstoppable fat burning force!

By combining both of these diets, you'll be able to take advantage of the strong points of both diets, have them counteract each other's weaknesses, and best of all stay lean for life!

Chapter 1: Why the Struggle is Real With Weight Loss

The first time I wanted to burn body fat and get ripped six pack abs was when I was 16 years old. I got my inspiration when I started watching fitness videos on the web, and saw impressive physiques that I wanted to emulate. I did what any normal person would do, and I went all out in order to achieve my goal as soon as possible.

- I immediately cut out all of the junk food from my diet.
- I ate 6 small meals a day, none of which exceeded 250 calories.
- I wouldn't eat anything that contained more than 10% of the total calories from fat.
- I would workout multiple times a day, 6 days per week.
- I would drink a gallon of water a day (of course from a gallon milk jug).
- I even refused to eat my own birthday cake—that's how dedicated I was!

Of course, everything was going smoothly at first. I was so motivated and dedicated that nothing was going to come in my way and stop me. Then it happened. I was doing another one of my intense six-pack ab workouts in my garage. I was low on calories, and I was working out in a place with no air conditioning in the Texas summer heat. I ended up nearly blacking out and having to quit my workout because I felt like I was going to pass out.

And I'm not the type of guy to quit right in the middle of a workout, so I felt very guilty for giving up. I later came to my senses and realized that this wasn't a sustainable approach to getting in shape. Sure, I was starting to notice some progress, but it came at the cost of me having to be a slave to my fitness routine. My whole life revolved around fitness!

I came to realize an important lesson on that day—**the point of health and fitness is to enhance your life, not control it.**

I'm sure you can relate to my story. Whenever we want something, we want it now! And that type of mentality causes us to do crazy things we normally wouldn't. For me, it was crash dieting and working out too much, and for you it might be something similar. The point is that we have to slow down and realize that weight loss is a marathon and not a sprint.

Too many people treat weight loss like a 100-yard dash and that's why they crash and burn like I did. Instead you must focus on the bigger overall picture and learn how to better pace yourself like a marathon runner would do. Yes, every decision you make in regards to diet and exercise matters, however no single choice will completely ruin you.

Eating a cookie for example, isn't a big deal in the grand scheme of things. However, if you eat a cookie, feel guilty for doing it, and then proceed to say "screw it" and binge eat, you've made the problem much worse than it ever was.

You will mess up and fall off track at times and that's ok as long as you get back up and keep going. Understanding this from the start is key because you can still fail, even if you have a solid nutrition plan in place like the fasting keto diet. Let's say for example, you have a sprinter's mindset with the fasting keto diet. You'll still cut your overall calories lower than you're supposed to, and you'll want to quit once you make a mistake.

We're all human here, so mistakes will happen! When have you ever been perfect at something and failed to make a single mistake? The goal with the fasting keto diet isn't to be spot on 100% of the time, instead it's more important to be consistent roughly 85% of the time. This will not only take a lot of pressure off of you for looming mishaps, but you'll still be able to obtain amazing results for a long time to come!

Chapter 2: What is Fasting?

Intermittent fasting is simply taking a break from eating for a prolonged period of time. I'll get into the different styles of fasting that exist in a bit, but for now know this—when you fast, you don't eat. It really is that simple, and that's one of the many reasons why I enjoy intermittent fasting so much. There are also no specific foods that are forbidden for you to eat when you're not fasting.

This makes fasting a very flexible type of diet—so flexible in fact, that it can easily be paired with other diet strategies, such as the ketogenic diet (more on that later). Every diet that has ever been created is designed to put you into a caloric deficit (I'll be covering what that is later on) one way or another.

For example, a low fat diet will reduce overall calories by reducing fat intake. Going on a diet consisting of nothing but healthy foods will try to achieve the same goal by eliminating high calorie junk food items. Fasting is no different, and its main way of getting you into a caloric deficit will be by reducing meal frequency.

Unlike eating low fat foods or eating healthy 24/7, you'll actually be able to fast for a long time to come. Not only that, but it's also an enjoyable nutrition plan once you get used to it! Many diet plans are very boring and make you eat bland foods like chicken breast and broccoli all of the time.

These were some of the things that originally got me interested in fasting back when I first started it. However, I quickly came to learn a couple of things:

1. The first couple of weeks can be pretty tough as your body starts to adapt to fasting.
2. The method of fasting you do is critically important to ensure a good fit with your schedule and lifestyle. You'll have to test various styles out to see what works best for you.

For myself, I originally started fasting with Brad Pilon's *Eat Stop Eat* method. I'll cover more details on this fasting method later, but all you need to know for now is that it involves a 24-hour fast, 1-2 days per week. This method works great for a lot of people, but it didn't work that great for me. I found it too hard to get in a good rhythm with fasting because I was only fasting twice per week. I needed something that involved a more consistent fast.

I eventually found a fasting method that worked for me, and it was so easy to maintain that I was able to do intermittent fasting for years without a problem. (I'll share what it was in the following chapter.) The main point is that different people have different schedules, bodies, lifestyles, etc.—therefore, it's important to realize that, although one fasting method did/didn't work for me, it doesn't mean that method won't work for you.

Chapter 3: Different Methods of Fasting

Now it's time for the fun part. How exactly do you fast? Do you fast as long as you want and call it a day? Should you fast all day?

How often should you fast? As it turns out, there are quite a few different styles of fasting that exist. I'll share with you the pros and cons of each, and I'll tell you which method worked the best for me in terms of long-term sustainability.

Fasting Method #1: The Warrior Diet

Ori Hofmekler created this style of fasting, and it involves a monstrous 20-hour daily fast and a 4-hour feeding window. This is definitely on the extreme end considering you'll be fasting for about 83% of the time in a day. You'll eat small amounts of fruits and vegetables during the day.

Then at night you'll get to enjoy a large feast. You can eat to your heart's content during your meal. It's unlikely that you'll overeat your allotted calories during one meal.

Typical number of meals per day: 1

Pros of the Warrior Diet:

-Easy way to ensure fat loss because it's unlikely you'll overeat from 1 meal.
-You'll get to enjoy a large amount of calories in 1 meal.
-You can enjoy eating your favorite foods with little worry of overeating.

Cons of the Warrior Diet:

-It's tough. Fasting for 20 hours a day can be hard to get used to.
-Not a flexible diet. Imagine your coworkers want you to come grab lunch with them. You can't go. Or maybe there's a birthday party you go to one weekend afternoon. You can't eat at the party. All of your social events must revolve around that 4-hour feeding window. Since that period of time is so small, it's unlikely to happen. You'll be forced to either cheat on your nutrition plan, or be "that guy" who's too good to eat at a party.

Fasting Method #2: Eat Stop Eat

Brad Pilon is the inventor of this style of fasting, and it involves doing a 24-hour fast 1-2 times per week. The main goal with this is to reduce your total caloric intake by 10-15% through fasting. The rest of the time, you'll eat as you normally would.

For example, let's say you're going to do a 24-hour fast on a Wednesday and you start the fast at noon. You won't be able to eat anything until noon on Thursday. The key is to sleep during the hardest part of the fast. So if you notice you get really hungry after fasting for 12 hours, time it to where you go to sleep around the 12-hour mark.

Typical number of meals per day: 3

Pros of Eat Stop Eat:

-Easy way to control calories once you adapt to it.
-This method allows you to eat as you normally would when you're not fasting.
-Flexible enough to allow you to choose when you want to start the fast.
-You can sleep during the hardest part of the fast.

Cons of Eat Stop Eat:

-Can be hard to adapt to since you're only fasting 1-2 days per week and the fast is for 24 hours.
-Can be intrusive to your life on days that you fast. For example, you can't eat with friends or family on days you fast and working around this often can be tough.

Fasting Method #3: The 5:2 Diet

This method of fasting is similar to Eat Stop Eat. Popularized by Michael Mosley, this nutrition plan involves eating as you normally would 5 days of the week and only eating 500-600 calories on the other 2 days. For example, you would eat as you normally would every day except for Tuesday and Friday. On these days you would eat two small meals of around 250 calories each for women and 300 for men.

Typical number of meals per day: 3 on non-fasting days, 2 on fasting days

Pros of the 5:2 Diet:

-This plan allows you to start losing weight without changing any of the foods you typically eat.
-You get to eat two small meals on fasting days whenever you want. This provides you with *some* flexibility to eat with friends and family.
-You'll be eating the way you normally do the majority of the time.

Cons of The 5:2 Diet

-You fast infrequently (only two days per week) making it hard to adapt to.
-There's a drastic difference between days when you fast and days you don't fast, making it hard to get used to.
-It's possible to be social and eat with friends on fasting days, but the possibility of overeating during these meals is high.

Fasting Method #4: Fasting Every Other Day

This is an extreme method of fasting that involves fasting every other day. You'll eat as you normally would one day, and then fast the next day. There are different variations to this style of fasting that allow you to eat 500 calories on your fasting days. If you can pull it off, you'll definitely see some results; it's unlikely you'll overeat from only consuming calories 3-4 days per week.

Typical number of meals per day: 3 on non-fasting days, 0 on fasting days

Pros of Fasting Every Other Day

-Very likely to see weight loss results.
-You can eat as you normally would during non-fasting days.

Cons of Fasting Every Other Day

-Not for beginners. Don't try it if you've never done fasting before.
-Too extreme for most people to handle.
-Frequent fasting makes it difficult to enjoy social meals with friends and family.
-Not necessary to start seeing results.

Fasting Method #5: The Leangains Method

Mark Berkhan popularized this style of fasting and it involves a daily fast of 16 hours and a feeding window of 8 hours. Typically, you'll eat 3 meals every 4 hours. For example, let's say your last meal of the day was at 8 p.m. You would fast until noon the next day and have meals at the following times:

Meal #1: Noon
Meal #2: 4:00 p.m.
Meal #3: 8:00 p.m.

Essentially what this boils down to is skipping breakfast. Yes, it'll take some time to adapt to this style of eating, but it fits in seamlessly with most lifestyles.

Typical number of meals per day: 3

Pros of Leangains:

-Daily fasting makes it easy to stick to once you get used to it.
-You're only skipping breakfast, which isn't a meal you typically eat with friends anyway.
-You still get to consume 3 meals a day.
-Fairly effortless and easy way to control calories.

Cons of Leangains
-More flexibility than most fasting methods, but it could still do better. For example, what do you do if you stay up late one night until 2 a.m.? You wouldn't be allowed to eat anything past 8 p.m. using the schedule from above. Wouldn't it be better if you could eat at 2 a.m. and start your next fast from there?

Fasting Method #6: Flex Fasting

Who popularized flex fasting? No one. It's a name I made up for this style of fasting because it sounds cool. Flex fasting is a modified version of the Leangains method of fasting, and it's the method I used to get great results with fasting.

Instead of having a strict 16-hour fast and 8 hour feeding window, you'll simply push your first meal of the day back 4-5 hours after you wake up. It doesn't matter when your last meal of the day is, or what time you go to bed at. All you need to do is follow one simple rule—wake up and don't eat for at least 4-5 hours. For example, if you wake up at 8:00 a.m., don't eat anything until noon or 1:00 p.m.

Sometimes you'll only end up fasting for 12 hours, and other times you'll fast for up to 18 hours. Generally, you'll hover around the 14-16 hour mark and that's great. The main idea isn't to have some strict amount of time you have to fast for. The key is to have flexibility.

This way you can enjoy life *while* you lose weight. You're in control of your diet, and your diet no longer calls the shots. Think about it. Most diets give you specific times and boring foods you must eat at those times.

It doesn't matter if you're hungry, or if you're in the mood to eat those foods. You must do it to lose weight. Your life must revolve around fitness in order for it to work. Most people realize it isn't worth it (because it's definitely not) and they quit.

Fortunately, flex fasting gives you a better option. Yes, I'm biased towards this fasting method, but remember, *all* of the fasting methods outlined here will work. You have to pick which one you think will work best for you and try it out. You'll never know until you give it a shot.

I've personally been doing fasting for about four years now and I've tried many different methods. During my first two years of fasting, I flip flopped between many of the different styles, and I never found one that was a homerun for me. Then I started doing flex fasting, and it has by far been the easiest method for me to stick with. It fits in seamlessly with my life.

I don't get crazy hungry because I have to fast 20 hours a day or anything like that. It has the best balance between structure and flexibility, which is why I recommend trying it for yourself.

Typical number of meals per day: 3

Pros of Flex Fasting:

-Extremely flexible for most schedules.
-Easy and effortless way to control calories.
-Will allow you to still be able to eat social meals with friends.

Cons of Flex Fasting:

-Lacks rigid structure. This makes it easy to bend the rules or not follow them at all.

Fasting Method #7: Skip Meals When Convenient

This last method isn't a structured fasting protocol like the previous ones are. It simply involves you skipping meals when it's convenient to do so or when you're not hungry. This gives you maximum flexibility, but the complete lack of structure will make it difficult to obtain any lasting results.

How often do we get around to doing something when it's convenient? Hardly ever because when it's not convenient to do something, we'll delay taking action.

Typical number of meals per day: 1-3

Pros of Skipping Meals When Convenient

-Provides maximum flexibility allowing for seamless fit into any lifestyle or schedule.
-Easy nutrition plan to get started with—simply start skipping meals when you can.

Cons of Skipping Meals When Convenient

-Lacks structure making it easy to not take any action.
-Unlikely to provide any results because you're only skipping meals when you feel like it, which will be few and far between.

Pick One and Get Started

Now that you know the different methods of fasting, the main thing is to get started. Choose the style you think will work best for you and try it out. If you're not sure which one to pick, start with method #6—flex fasting. Be sure to test it out for 2 weeks before moving on to a different method. Don't let all of the different choices paralyze you into not taking action. If you've never done fasting before, you won't know what works best for you until you start testing the choices out.

Chapter 4: History and Benefits of Fasting

Fasting is a great diet to get and stay in shape, and its benefits can even be combined with the benefits of the ketogenic diet for an even more powerful effect. The cool thing about fasting (and the ketogenic diet for that matter) is that our ancestors ate that way whether they realized it or not, so fasting certainly isn't a new idea, even though it has gained popularity in recent times. People have been fasting for thousands of years for various reasons—religious purposes, preparing for war, political protests, healing of illnesses (before medicine became prevalent), and even out of necessity.

Muslims fast while the sun is up during the month of Ramadan. Roman Catholics fast for 40 days during Lent to represent the 40 days Jesus fasted in the desert. Judaism has several annual fasts as well. Fasting was sometimes demanded before going to war as part of a ritual. And figures like Mahatma Gandhi have fasted for 21 days straight during the struggle for Indian independence.

It wasn't until recently that people began fasting for the enhanced health and fat loss benefits. Imagine for a second that you're a nomadic hunter and gather living thousands of years ago. Every day when you wake up, you can't simply go to the fridge and get something to eat. You must earn your food for the day by hunting for it.

Therefore, a lot of hunters had to fast because there wasn't anything to eat in the morning. Fast-forward to the present day and things are much different. Today, there's an overabundance of food. Anytime you want, you can drive through a 24/7 fast food restaurant and get something to eat.

You don't have to burn calories hunting for your food; you get in your car and drive to go get it. This is part of the reason why there is an obesity epidemic in America. Yes, having convenient restaurants and grocery stores is awesome, but they come at a price.

We're no longer forced to delay eating or have to earn it with exercise. How many people tell themselves, "I'll only eat this burger if I exercise for 30 minutes," or, "I'll eat this burger for lunch, but I won't eat anything else until then so I don't overeat." No one does this! It's easier to eat the burger now and worry about the consequences later.

Are We Even Meant to Eat Breakfast Anyway?

You've undoubtedly heard things before like, "Breakfast is the most important meal of the day," or, "Start your day off right with a good balanced breakfast." But were we even meant to eat breakfast anyway? Our ancestors didn't eat breakfast.

They had to wake up and hunt for their food. They didn't have an endless amount of cereal and pastries at their fingertips right when they woke up. So what happened? It wasn't until the 15th century that the word breakfast came into use in written English to describe a morning meal.

So the idea of breakfast has been around for quite some time, but it wasn't until recently that it became popularized. It all started with two men, Will Keith Kellogg and C.W. Post, creating their own cereal companies—Kellogg Company and Postum Cereal Company (now known as Post Cereals). The key to these companies' success came down to two factors—sugar and marketing.

Thanks to a barrage of advertising, cereal was able to maintain a reputation that it was a healthy food. It would even go as far as to claim that cereal cured everything up to malaria and appendicitis. This was even the start of claims such as, "a good source of Vitamin D!"

And to appeal to children, companies created cartoon mascots such as Tony the Tiger and Snap, Crackle, and Pop, which started appearing around the 1930s. Finally, there's the phrase, "Breakfast is the most important meal of the day." Cereal companies must first convince you to eat breakfast, and then get you to buy their cereal.

If they can do that, then they're in the clear because most people eat the same thing for breakfast everyday. Additionally, cereal was fast and convenient to make, which became increasingly important as corporate America was developing in the industrial age. Breakfast is a meal just like lunch or dinner. And while it may not be the most important, it certainly is the most marketed meal of the three.

Benefits of Fasting

Aside from making fat loss a breeze, what else can you expect to gain from a fasting nutrition plan? Quite a few things as it turns out...

-Live a longer life: There is evidence to suggest that fasting can help improve lifespan (1).

-Your body will become more efficient at using fat for fuel (2): When you fast, your body becomes glycogen depleted. Your body will then use fat stores for energy, and therefore learn to use fat for fuel for more effectively.

-Fasting can help to improve cognitive brain function, which will help to improve learning (3).

-Increased human growth hormone levels (hgh) (4): HGH is an important hormone for developing a lean and muscular body. It's responsible for muscle and bone growth, regulation of fluids, and regulation of body composition.

-You'll save time and money: Think about it. You won't have to spend as much time preparing, cooking, and eating meals. Plus, you'll save money at the grocery store!

-Improve focus and concentration: Have you ever felt sluggish or sleepy after eating a meal? The reason is because carbs make tryptophan more accessible to the brain. The tryptophan gets converted into serotonin, which eventually turns into melatonin. Melatonin regulates sleep and increases drowsiness. Therefore, by skipping breakfast you'll be more alert and focused, allowing you to be more productive in the morning.

-Faster recovery from sickness: There is evidence to suggest that fasting can help the body save energy and reduce heat loss, thus allowing it to focus solely on fighting off infection (5).

-Fasting may have positive effects on insulin resistance, thus reducing risk for type 2 diabetes (6).

-Fasting can help to reduce total cholesterol, blood pressure, and triglycerides (7).

Chapter 5: What is the Ketogenic Diet?

The ketogenic diet is a low-carb, high-fat, and moderate protein diet. The main premise behind the diet is to make your body more efficient at using fat for fuel instead of sugar. When you're consuming a lot of carbohydrates, your body's blood sugar levels will spike up. Your body will then release a hormone called insulin to help regulate your blood sugar back down to normal. Here are the two main functions of insulin:

1. To tell fat cells to produce and store fat, and to hold on to the fat they already carry.
2. To pick up glucose from the bloodstream and burn that glucose instead of fat.

What it boils down to is that insulin fuels lipolysis, which is the burning of fat; insulin also fuels lipogenesis, which is the production of fat. Needless to say, insulin is very important to be in control of if you want to burn fat! Remember, the second function of insulin is to burn off glucose in the bloodstream instead of fat. This means that if you're eating a lot of carbs, your body will be focusing on burning off those carbs rather than fat. Unfortunately, your body doesn't burn *any* fat when insulin levels are spiked (8).

This makes sense because carbs are your body's first source of energy (9), so it'll tap into that first and then go to your fat stores. Of course, that's not what we want! In a perfect world, we would get to choose for our bodies to use fat for fuel as its first source of energy, but sadly it doesn't work that way. Instead, we must keep our insulin levels low by lowering our carbohydrate intake, and then our bodies will be forced to burn fat for fuel instead of carbs.

Luckily, this is where the ketogenic diet really shines. By following a ketogenic diet, you'll lower your carbs enough to put your body in a metabolic state known as ketosis. When you're in a state of ketosis, your body becomes way more efficient at burning fat for fuel instead of carbohydrates (10). The name of the game with the ketogenic diet is to stay in a state of ketosis for as long as you can!

Different Ways to Do the Ketogenic Diet

Believe it or not, there are actually quite a few different ways out there you can do the ketogenic diet based on your individual needs:

Standard Ketogenic Diet: this is the most common and most popular version of the ketogenic diet, and it's the one we'll mostly be focusing on. It involves consuming around 75% of your calories from fat, 20% from protein, and the remaining 5% from carbs.

Targeted Ketogenic Diet: with this type of ketogenic diet, you'll add in carbs before and after your workouts. Other than that, everything else is the same as the standard keto diet. Typically you'll consume around .33 grams of carbs per pound of bodyweight before and after your workout. For most people, this will equate to roughly 40-80 grams of carbs per meal. Pre and post workout carbohydrates have been shown to increase performance and aid in recovery (11). Therefore, if you're an athlete or an individual who trains with a lot of intensity on a regular basis, this type of ketogenic diet is for you.

Cyclical Ketogenic Diet: this is more of an advanced type of ketogenic diet. With this style of keto, you'll devote one or two full days to eating high carbohydrates in order to refill muscle glycogen stores. You'll usually consume around 50%

of your total calories from carbs on these days. This will help to promote muscle growth for athletes or individuals looking to build muscle. A proper workout routine (which will be covered later) must be in place in order for you to fully deplete your muscle glycogen stores. If not, you could end up gaining a little bit of body fat. Due to the precise planning and fact that's it's easy to overeat on your high-carb days, this version of keto isn't recommended for beginners.

High-Protein Ketogenic Diet: this style of ketogenic diet is similar to the standard ketogenic diet, except that it contains more protein and less fat. Typically you'll eat around 60% fat, 35% protein, and 5% carbs with this type of ketogenic diet. This style is great for individuals who engage regularly in vigorous activity and want a higher protein intake to help prevent muscle loss. Protein is also very satiating and will help to keep you fuller for a longer period of time when your calories are being restricted.

For the purposes of this book, we'll be focusing our attention mostly on the standard ketogenic diet. This version of the ketogenic diet is backed by the most research and it's the easiest for beginners to get started with.

Foods to Avoid:

Eating low carbs might seem easy enough to do on the surface, but many people struggle with knowing exactly what constitutes a low-carb food vs. a high-carb food. Carbs are contained in many different foods that you may not realize. The best thing you can do if you're unsure is to look it up online and see how many carbs a certain food actually contains.

Later on, I'll be providing you with some keto friendly recipes that you can use while on the diet. For now however, I want to provide you with a list of foods that you'll need to avoid eating while on the ketogenic diet. These are foods that are high in sugar or carbs and will take you out of ketosis. Here's the list:

Grains: any wheat-based product such as rice, cereal, pasta, etc.

Fruit: yes fruit is healthy for you, however for the purposes of the ketogenic diet it's not allowed because fruit contains fructose and that will take your body out of ketosis.

Sugary foods: this would include things such as fruit juice, smoothies, ice cream, cookies, candy, soda, diet soda, and other sugar-free diet foods. Sugar-free foods usually contain sugar alcohols, which can affect ketone levels.

Alcohol: alcoholic drinks contain a high amount of carbs and can kick you out of ketosis.

Unhealthy fats: yes, the ketogenic diet is a high fat diet, however you want to be consuming healthy fats. Avoid processed vegetable oils and trans fat.

Low-Fat products: many low-fat food items are either high in sugar or carbs to replace the fat content and should be avoided.

Beans: yes most beans are healthy, but the high-carb content will ruin the benefits of the diet. Avoid eating any type of bean including: peas, lentils, chickpeas, black beans, kidney beans, etc.

Root Vegetables: you might be thinking, "What? I thought vegetables were good for you!" Yes, vegetables certainly are good for you, but particular vegetables are higher in carbs and will do more harm than good while on a ketogenic diet. Don't consume potatoes, sweet potatoes, carrots, turnips, etc.

Foods to Eat

The list of foods to avoid is quite large, and it might leave you wondering what you can eat on a ketogenic diet. Luckily, there are still plenty of foods you can eat that will provide plenty of variety so you'll never get bored constantly eating the same foods over and over:

Eggs: eggs are a great source of protein and fat, and they contain no carbs. It's a versatile food that can be made in a lot of different dishes.

Cheese: cheese gets a bad rep for being unhealthy, but it's a very keto-friendly food. It contains virtually no carbs and will help you reach your daily fat intake.

Nuts: various nuts such as almonds, cashews, peanuts, etc. contain healthy fats and are a great snack choice if you're on the go a lot.

Seeds: pumpkin seeds, chia seeds, flaxseeds, etc. are high in fiber and can easily be thrown into many dishes without changing the taste of the recipe.

Healthy Oils: similar to seeds, healthy oils such as olive oil and coconut oil can be added seamlessly to dishes without a noticeable difference in taste.

Low-Carb Vegetables: not all vegetables are excluded from the ketogenic diet. Any leafy green vegetable can be eaten along with onions and peppers without worry of exceeding your carb limit.

Butter: Similar to cheese, butter tends to get labeled as unhealthy. However, when it comes to butter, the quality and kind you get matters big time. Stay away from the margarine and buy grass-fed if you can.

Avocados: makes for great guacamole and avocados are a healthy fat. Enough said.

Chapter 6: Health Benefits of the Ketogenic Diet

Research has shown the ketogenic diet to be a great way to lose weight (12). That's cool and all, but losing weight shouldn't be the only thing you seek with a diet. You should have more energy, and better indications of health such as lower cholesterol. Starting a ketogenic diet can provide you with some amazing health benefits in addition to losing weight:

Prevention of diabetes: diabetes is essentially an impaired function of insulin. Studies have shown the ketogenic diet to be able to improve insulin sensitivity (13). The higher your insulin sensitivity levels are, the less insulin your body will require to lower blood glucose levels back to normal. As you learned in the previous chapter, your body doesn't burn fat when insulin levels are high. Therefore, it's important to improve insulin sensitivity levels to help better regulate blood glucose levels.

Lower Risk for Heart disease: heart disease is one of the leading causes of death in the United States, and it includes many risk factors such as cholesterol levels, body fat, blood sugar, and blood pressure. The ketogenic diet can help to improve these risk factors, thus lowering the risk for heart disease (14).

Getting rid of acne: another cool side benefit is that it can help get rid of acne if you struggle with breakouts regularly. The ketogenic diet will help to lower insulin levels by eating less processed foods and sugar, which can help prevent acne.

Cancer treatment: the ketogenic diet is currently being used to treat several different types of cancer, and it can slow tumor growth (15). Of course, more research needs to be done for conclusive evidence.

Increase HDL cholesterol levels: there are two different kinds of cholesterol—HDL, which stands for high-density lipoproteins and LDL, which stands for low-density lipoproteins. Your HDL is your good cholesterol that you want to increase because it's responsible for carrying cholesterol to the liver where it can then be excreted or reused. LDL's on the other hand, are bad cholesterol, and are responsible for carrying cholesterol away from the liver and into the body. Research shows one of the best ways to increase your HDL levels are to increase your fat intake (16). You'll easily be able to achieve that with the standard ketogenic protocol of 75% of your calories coming from fat.

Lower blood pressure: Lowering your carbohydrate intake has been shown to decrease hypertension (17). Having higher blood pressure increases your risk for developing diseases such as heart disease and stroke.

Decrease triglyceride levels: triglycerides are a fat molecule. It might sound counter-intuitive that increasing your fat intake would decrease the amount of triglycerides in the blood, but it really does. This occurs because carbs are one of the biggest contributors to increasing triglycerides (18). Therefore, by decreasing carb intake, you'll decrease the amount of triglycerides in your blood.

More weight loss than a typical diet: Studies have shown that people who restrict calories on a low-carb diet lose more weight, and lose weight faster than individuals restricting calories on a low-fat diet (19). The main reason for this is because low-carb diets lower insulin levels, which will cause the body to get rid of excess sodium within the first few weeks of starting the diet.

A positive way to lose your appetite: When you go on a diet and restrict your calories, you start to feel hungry. If your feelings of hunger start to get out of control, you're more likely to quit and give up on your diet—and obviously if you quit and go back to your old habits, you have no chance of losing weight and improving your health. Luckily, eating a low-carb diet has been shown to decrease appetite (20). This is critical because it'll allow you to lower your overall caloric intake without having to worry about getting extra hungry.

Chapter 7: Why Combine Fasting with the Ketogenic Diet?

When I first started working out, I wanted to achieve all of my fitness goals at once:

- Get a six-pack
- Dunk a basketball
- Build muscle
- Run faster
- Increase endurance

And by chasing all of these rabbit holes, I ended up achieving none of my goals. Looking back on it, I realized that it's better to focus on achieving one goal at a time before moving onto the next. In my case, I would need to dunk a basketball before moving onto trying to lean down to get a six-pack. Then, once I got ripped six-pack abs, I would then try to accomplish another goal such as increasing endurance.

Why then should you try to combine fasting with the ketogenic diet? Won't you be spreading yourself too thin and end up not achieving anything like I did when I first started working out? The answer is no because intermittent fasting and the ketogenic diet work synergistically together to achieve one common goal—fat loss. My problem was that I wanted to achieve varying goals that contrasted one another.

For example, I wanted to build muscle and burn fat at the same time. Yes, this is possible for beginners to pull off, but it usually complicates things. This is because in order for you to build muscle, you need to be in a caloric surplus by consuming more calories than you burn off. And in order for you to burn fat, you need to be in a caloric deficit by burning off more calories than you consume (I'll go more in depth on surpluses and deficits later). Since you can't be in a surplus and a deficit at the same time, can you see how these contradictory goals can complicate things?

I tried heading in one direction to build muscle, and then I would turn around and go in the opposite direction to try and burn fat. In the end, I stayed exactly where I was at and went nowhere. Keep things simple and go for one goal at a time. Lose all of the weight that you want, and then start trying to build muscle.

Fortunately, it's easy to combine fasting with the ketogenic diet to maximize the health and weight loss benefits. All you'll need to do is find a fasting method from chapter 3 that works best for you. Once you're comfortable with fasting, you'll simply eat a ketogenic diet within your eating window of the intermittent fasting diet. For example, let's say you decide to implement the lean gains method of fasting where you'll fast for 16 hours a day and eat during the remaining 8 hours of the day.

You might eat meals during these times of the day:

Meal #1: Noon
Meal #2: 4:00 p.m.
Meal #3: 8:00 p.m.

When you eat each of those three meals, you'll eat a low-carb, high fat keto type of meal. This works perfectly because one of the most common questions people have with intermittent fasting is, "What should I eat?" Fasting doesn't provide much structure for what to eat, but luckily the ketogenic diet makes up for that weakness. You have structure with each meal you eat because you know it has to contain a very low amount of carbs, a high amount of fat, and a moderate amount of protein. There are also many different recipes you can follow for ideas of what to eat.

Conversely, the ketogenic doesn't do a good job of telling you *when* to eat. It can be all over the place. Do you eat a standard breakfast, lunch, and dinner? Are you allowed to have snacks? Can you eat as frequently as you want? Fortunately, intermittent fasting will cover up this weakness of the ketogenic diet. Your fasting protocol will tell you when you can and cannot eat. It helps to keep things simple. During your fast, no snacks are allowed. And the fasting method you choose will determine how many meals per day you eat.

For example, with the Warrior Diet style of fasting, you'll only eat one meal per day. And with the 5:2 diet, you'll eat 2-3 small meals on your fasting days. Ultimately, you'll have to test different fasting methods with the ketogenic diet to see what works best for your individual schedule and lifestyle.

Chapter 8: Setting Up & Executing Your Fasting Keto Diet

Here's the exact step-by-step process you need to take to set up your fasting keto diet:

Step #1: Understand the Importance of Calories

You've undoubtedly heard of the word calorie before. But what exactly is a calorie? Is it something evil you should avoid whenever possible? Is it the bane of your existence?

Many people have an idea of what a calorie is, but most don't know. If you went out on the street and asked ten different people what a calorie is, you'd likely get ten different answers. Here's the textbook definition of a calorie:

"The energy needed to raise the temperature of 1 gram of water through 1° C"

Sounds complicated right? Essentially, a calorie is a measurement of energy. Your body is constantly undergoing chemical reactions to keep you alive. All of these chemical reactions (digestion, breathing, organ function, etc.) require energy.

Your body gets the energy necessary to continue functioning from the food (calories) you eat. Calories aren't your worst enemy; they're your friend. You have to work with them, not against them. And as you're about to find out, not all calories are the same.

Is a Calorie a Calorie?

This is a big debate in the fitness industry. If I eat 100 calories from a candy bar, and you eat 100 calories worth of vegetables, are we equal? Well, yes and no.

One calorie *is* one calorie regardless of what source the calorie came from. Trying to argue with this is like saying one yard going east isn't the same distance as going one yard west. The difference lies in the *macronutrient* quality.

100 calories from vegetables and 100 calories from candy is still 100 calories. Both are made up mostly of carbs; the quality of those carbs is what makes them very different. The candy contains simple carbs and sugar.

It won't provide you with any vitamins, nutrients, or fiber. It also won't be very satiating. The vegetables, on the other hand, are complex carbs.

They'll provide you with quality complex carbs and a good source of vitamins, nutrients, and fiber. Additionally, nutritious food like fruits and vegetables will keep you fuller longer, which is critical during calorie restriction for weight loss purposes. Therefore, quality of calories can be just as important as quantity of calories.

The Caloric Deficit is King

Pop quiz: What's the *only* way your body can burn fat?

If you looked at the title above and guessed caloric deficit, then you'd be correct! A caloric deficit is simply when you burn off more calories than you consume. The opposite is a caloric surplus—consuming more calories than you burn off. And maintenance is when you are at a caloric equilibrium.

Here's an example:

-Joe burns 2,000 calories a day and eats 1,800. He's in a caloric deficit of 200 calories and he'll start to lose weight.
-Joe burns 2,000 calories a day and eats 2,200. He's in a caloric surplus of 200 calories and he'll start to gain weight.
-Joe burns 2,000 calories a day and eats 2,000. He's at maintenance and will not gain or lose weight.

Starting a fasting keto diet isn't enough to guarantee results. It's still possible for you to overeat on healthy fats and not lose any weight. It's also possible for you to eat too little and crash and burn because you're hungry all of the time. That's why you must know the numbers behind exactly how much you need to eat in order to lose weight. The fasting keto diet will structure *how* you eat, but determining your resting metabolic rate in the next step will determine the *amount* you need to eat to start burning fat.

Step #2: Determine Your Resting Metabolic Rate

As I mentioned earlier, every day your body needs energy (calories) in order to continue on with all of its chemical functions like breathing, digesting food, organ function, etc. The amount of calories you burn in any given day is your resting metabolic rate (rmr). Once you figure out your body's rmr, you can then determine how many calories you need to eat to start burning fat.

Determining your rmr is simple—multiply your bodyweight in pounds by 13.
Let's use myself as an example:

Bodyweight=200 pounds
200 x 13= RMR of 2,600

This means that if I eat less than 2,600 calories, I'll be in a caloric deficit and I'll start to lose weight. If I eat more than 2,600 calories, I'll be in a caloric surplus and I'll start to gain weight. And finally, if I eat exactly 2,600 calories, I'll be at maintenance and I'll neither gain nor lose weight.

The question is—how big of a caloric deficit do you need to create in order for it to translate into pounds lost? There's about 3,500 calories in one pound of fat (21), meaning that you must create a cumulative caloric deficit of 3,500 calories in order to lose 1 pound. So if you divide 3,500 by 7 days in a week, you'll need to create an average daily caloric deficit of 500 calories to lose 1 pound per week.

Referring back to the example from above, here's what that would translate to:

RMR- 2,600 – 500= 2,100

This means that I need to eat 2,100 calories everyday if I want to lose 1 pound per week. The more weight you have to lose, the larger the caloric deficit you can create. For example, you could eat at a caloric deficit of 750 calories and lose 1.5 pounds per week, or you could eat at a deficit of 1,000 calories to lose 2 pounds per week.

Essentially, for every 250 calories you can expect to lose an additional .5-pound. The key is to not get carried away. You might want to lose all of the weight as soon as possible and jump right into a 1,000-calorie caloric deficit.

That may not be the best idea. For most people, losing 1 pound per week by creating a 500-calorie caloric deficit is golden. Imagine yourself a year from now being 52 pounds lighter without having to put forth much effort! That's much better than spinning your wheels trying to lose 100 pounds in that same time frame.

Step #3: Set Up Your Macro Percentages

In case you're unfamiliar, a macro is simply a protein, carb, or fat. And now we're going to figure out exactly how many grams of carbs, protein, and fat you need to be eating on a daily basis. From there, you'll simply eat that much and start seeing results. It really is that simple.

Before we can get into the specifics of each macro, it's critical that you know what your resting metabolic rate is by multiplying your bodyweight by 13.

Then if you want to lose weight, subtract 500 from your RMR. This is the total amount of calories you'll eat on a daily basis.

Once you know that information, you can move onto the next section.

Setting Up Your Macro Percentages

The first thing we must determine is the percentage of our diet each macronutrient (protein, carb, and fat) will make up. Since we're following a standard ketogenic diet these are the percentages we'll use:

- Protein: 20% of total calories
- Carbs: 5% of total calories
- Fat: 75% of total calories

Now that you know the total amount of calories you need to eat, and you know the percentage for each macro, we can now determine how many calories of protein, carbs, and fat you'll need to eat. Before we do though, it's important to remember the following:

Number of calories per gram of protein=4
Number of calories per gram of carb=4
Number of calories per gram of fat=9

I'll use myself as an example again:

Resting metabolic rate=2,600 calories

If I want to burn fat:

2,600-500=2,100 daily calories

2,100 x .20= 420 total daily calories from protein
2,100 x .05= 105 total daily calories from carbs
2,100 x .75= 1,575 total daily calories from fat

You can determine the grams equivalent of these total calorie numbers by doing the following:

420/4=105 grams of protein per day
105/4=26.25 grams of carbs per day
1,575/9=175 grams of fat per day

Yes these numbers are very exact; however don't try to be perfect. The reality is that you'll rarely eat 26.25 grams of carbs spot on so don't fret over it. Instead, try to get within 5%-10% of the numbers and you'll be fine.

Step #4: Set Up Your Fasting Protocol

Once you have your macros setup, the next thing you need to do is implement your fasting protocol. You can choose from any of the fasting methods I mentioned in chapter 3, however some of them will fit better with the ketogenic part of the diet than others. For example, trying to mix the Warrior diet with the ketogenic diet could be disastrous.

This is because your calories are already being heavily restricted to one meal a day with the Warrior diet. Then on top of that, the only meal you get to eat will be low in carbs, which will further restrict your caloric intake. Eating that many grams of fat in one meal might be tough as well, making this an overall poor choice.

Start with a balanced fasting approach that'll easily work with the ketogenic diet. The two best methods are going to be either the Lean Gains method or the Flex Fasting method. Both of these styles involve shorter, but more frequent fasts. This way you'll be able to eat a normal number of meals per day (usually 3) that won't make you feel as if you're starving yourself.

Play around with the different styles and see what works best for you. If you have previous experience with the Eat Stop Eat style, for example, and you know it works for you, then go with that one. If you're completely new to fasting and the ketogenic diet, then I recommend that you focus solely on intermittent fasting for two weeks before adding in the ketogenic diet. This way you'll give your body time to adapt to this new style of eating before you move onto the next one.

You'll make things far easier on yourself instead of crashing and burning from trying to do too much at once. All you need to do during this two-week period is follow the fasting protocol as it's laid out. Don't worry about what to eat, only follow the guidelines of the fast. For example, if you're doing Lean Gains, fast for 16 hours a day and don't worry about what you're eating for those two weeks. The sole purpose of this period is to get your body used to one thing at a time.

Then, once the two-weeks is up, you can start using the overall diet that includes the calories, macros, fasting, and ketogenic diet.

Step #5: Add in the Ketogenic Diet

Once you've gotten used to intermittent fasting, it's now time for the fun part. You're going to add in the keto diet with the fasting diet you've already started. Feel free to choose from any of the types of the keto diet I mentioned in chapter 5.

However, I would recommend sticking with the standard ketogenic diet especially if you're a beginner. This will help to keep things simple, and the standard ketogenic diet is the easiest one to follow; it'll work best for the average individual who's looking to get fit. To start your standard ketogenic diet, all you'll need to do is follow the macro parameters of 75% fat, 5% carbs, and 20% protein. From there, eat foods and follow recipes based on the recommended food list from chapter 5 regarding the keto diet. Of course, that's not a comprehensive list, so feel free to look up any additional foods that are allowed on a ketogenic diet.

Step #6: Measure and Adjust

You might be thinking, this sounds great and all, but how do I actually track and measure my calories and macro percentages? This is certainly the most tedious part of any diet, but remember what gets measured gets managed. You must track and account for the calories you're eating, or else you'll have no clue what direction you're heading in.

The easiest way to track your macros is to go to the app store, type in macro tracker, and download one of the many apps that will track your macros. Most of the apps cost a couple of dollars, but that's a small price to pay. You can type in the food you're eating and it'll tell you how many calories are contained in the food and how much protein, carbs, and fat it has. Most of the apps even have a barcode scanner where you can take a picture of what you're eating and it'll automatically add the macros towards your daily numbers.

You'll have your phone on you wherever you go, so if you eat at a restaurant, for example, you can track the macros and calories right then and there. If you decide not to use an app, you'll have to track your macros using nutritional labels or by searching the nutritional information online. From there, you'll have to calculate the numbers yourself and record it on a note app or with pen and paper, which is certainly not ideal.

The more inconvenient something is to do, the less likely you are to stick with it. The fasting keto diet is a great nutritional plan, but only if you're able to keep up with it for the long haul. You want to keep things as simple and easy as possible—spend a couple of bucks and indulge in a macro tracking app to take the load off your shoulders. It'll pay for itself many times over.

The other thing you'll need to get is a food scale. You can get one of these on Amazon for around $11. This'll allow you to figure out the number of grams in the foods you're eating and calculate the macros from there.

Once you've been doing this diet for a while, you'll eventually start to get a feel for how you need to eat in order to lose weight. You'll know the general macro contents of the meals you regularly eat. You'll be able to do the eyeball test and guess roughly how many calories are in the foods you're eating.

This is a skill that'll come with time. Be patient and don't rush it because that's when you'll start overestimating your calories. Tracking everything as accurately as possible is the key to success with any nutritional approach that you do. Be diligent about your measuring, especially in the beginning, even though it's quite tedious.

It might take you a couple of weeks to get used to measuring and recording everything that you eat and drink. Be patient with yourself if it takes a few weeks for you to start seeing results. You'll get better and better with the process as time goes on. Nobody is a master at something the first time they do it.

One common question people have with this topic is how close do I have to be with my macro percentages and calories? The reality is that you'll never be 100% accurate with your numbers. Using the example from earlier, you'll never eat exactly 26.25 grams of carbs each day and that's ok. You'll want to aim to be within 5-10% of what I recommend. For example, one day you might intake 65% of your diet from fat and 30% from protein. It's not worth the extra stress of getting every little number exactly right—you'll drive yourself nuts. You want to generally be as consistent and accurate as you possibly can.

The other thing you'll want to do is measure your weight. One mistake a lot of people make is that they weigh themselves too often. Our bodies are constantly fluctuating in weight sometimes by as much as 5 pounds (22). So one morning you might weigh yourself and the scale says you lost weight so you're happy. Then the next day you step on the scale and now you gained half a pound.

At this point, you'd be freaking out and wondering, "What in the world is going on?" Imagine having to fight this psychological battle each and every week. Every week you have to overcome negative thoughts and worries:

- Is my diet actually working?
- Am I doing something wrong?
- Should I quit?
- Should I try a different nutritional approach?

You would have to overcome all of those doubts before you could start making any real progress. The reality is that nothing is wrong with you; the problem is that the scale is deceiving you. It's making you think that you've gained weight when in reality your bodyweight is simply fluctuating.

Therefore, it's important to weigh yourself as consistently as you possibly can. Weigh yourself first thing in the morning before you've eaten anything. In addition to that, only weigh yourself once a week. One week is long enough for you to know if the weight on the scale has gone down it's because of actual weight loss, not because of a fluctuation.

Overall, I want you to focus on the bigger picture when it comes to weight loss. Over the past 3 months, has the direction on the scale been going the way you want it to? If so, then great, you're making progress! That's what matters.

Don't freak out and question everything you're doing, all because you didn't lose any weight one week.

Chapter 9: How to Use Exercise to Maximize Fat Loss

The fasting keto diet is a great nutrition strategy, but you can also use it to help maximize fat loss in the gym. There are a couple of different ways to take advantage of this. The first way is by being in a fasted state when you workout. All you need to do is workout in the morning or early afternoon before you've eaten anything.

When you workout in a fed state, your body will use the glycogen in your body as fuel for energy. However when you workout fasted, your body will be glycogen depleted. This means that your body won't be able to tap into your glycogen stores for energy; it'll have to go somewhere else. Guess where that somewhere else is? Your fat stores!

By working out in a fasted state, your body will become more efficient at using fat for energy instead of carbs. The second thing you can do is delay eating after your workout. The media has done a good job of making us think we must immediately consume protein after a workout or else it was a waste. Research shows that your body won't lose muscle if you don't eat protein within 45 minutes of your workout (23).

Whenever you workout, your body's growth hormone levels will increase (24). This growth hormone will help to protect your muscle and increase fat burning. However, if you eat right after you finish a workout, your growth hormone levels will be blunted and insulin levels will increase. For this reason, you'll want to delay eating anything after finishing a workout for 1-2 hours.

Eating more calories won't help you lose more weight. Yet when it comes to eating after a workout, people act like they're immune to gaining fat from these extra calories. "I hit it hard in the gym today, I deserve a large milkshake!" No, you don't.

Imagine you go to the gym and burn 300 calories. Then, immediately after your workout, you consume a 350-calorie post workout protein shake. Now you've completely wiped out all of the calories you burned from the workout, plus you ate an additional 50 calories! It's ok to eat a meal after working out if that's when you would normally eat anyway.

Don't go out of your way to eat extra calories for the sake of a post workout shake—it won't help you burn more fat! You might be weary of working out fasted if you usually workout in a fed state. Give it a try for 1-2 weeks to give your body a chance to adapt to it. Once you do, you should notice that you have more focus and intensity in the gym.

Here's a good beginner's workout plan you can do if you're unsure of what to do in the gym:

This regimen consists of 3 full-body weight workouts per week. You'll complete the same workout every time you go to the gym. You can set up your workout schedule in one of the following ways:

Monday: Workout
Tuesday: Rest
Wednesday: Workout
Thursday: Rest
Friday: Workout
Saturday: Rest
Sunday: Rest

Or

Monday: Rest
Tuesday: Workout
Wednesday: Rest
Thursday: Rest
Friday: Rest
Saturday: Rest
Sunday: Rest

As a beginner, full-body workouts will provide you with many benefits:

-You'll burn more calories from your workouts.
-You'll gain strength and muscle faster since you'll be stimulating your muscles more frequently.
-You'll have better nervous system recovery because you won't train on consecutive days.
-You'll develop perfect form on key lifts faster because you practice them more often.

Essentially, your body has never been exposed to this stimulus (i.e. weightlifting) before. Therefore, you can take advantage of what some people call "newbie gains." By increasing the frequency at which you stimulate your muscle groups, you can speed up the process.

Side Note: A set is a group of consecutive repetitions. A repetition is one complete motion of an exercise. The rest period is how long of a break you'll take until you start the next set. For example, let's say you're completing 3 sets of 8 reps and resting 2 minutes in between sets for the barbell squat exercise.

You'll squat down and stand back up, completing the motion of the exercise and one rep. You'll repeat that motion 7 more times for a total of 8 repetitions. That will complete the set, and you will begin your rest period. Once your 2-minute rest period is up, you'll start the next set and perform another 8 repetitions.

That will complete set number 2, and you'll rest another 2 minutes. Once that time period is up, you'll complete the final set of 8 repetitions, and then you'll move onto the next exercise.

Here's the workout:

- Incline Barbell Bench Press: 3 sets 8 reps 2 min rest between (btw) sets
- Barbell Back Squats: 3 sets of 8 reps 2 min rest btw sets
- Lat Pulldowns: 3 sets of 10 reps 90 sec rest btw sets
- Seated DB Military Press: 3 sets of 8 reps 2 min rest btw sets
- Standing DB Curls: 3 sets of 12 reps 60 sec rest btw sets
- Tricep Rope Pushdowns: 3 sets of 12 reps 60 sec rest btw sets

That's all there is to it! Don't let the simplicity of it fool you—it will work.

What About Cardio?

If you're looking to burn fat, cardio can definitely be a handy tool to help you out. It's a great form of exercise you can do regardless if you're into weight training or not. Cardio will do one of two things for you:

#1: Speed up the rate at which you lose fat.

Or

#2: Give you some extra leeway in your diet.

Cardio is by no means necessary for you to reach your fat loss goals, but it will help. What type of cardio should you do—slow and steady or running? Science shows that the best type of cardio you can do is something called high intensity interval training (HIIT) (25).

This kind of cardio combines high intensity cardio with low intensity cardio. HIIT by itself is very effective, but it can be maximized when you immediately follow it with slow steady state cardio. The intensity of the HIIT will release free fatty acids into your bloodstream, and the slow steady state cardio will burn them off. Here's how to perform this hybrid cardio workout:

Part 1: HIIT

Alternate between a high intensity and a low intensity for 10-15 minutes on your choice of cardio machine. Here's an example on a treadmill:
-Run at 7.5 mph for 1 minute
-Walk at 3.5 mph for 1 minute
-Repeat for 10-15 minutes

Part 2: Slow steady state cardio (done immediately after HIIT)

Example on a treadmill: Walk at a constant pace of 3.5-4 mph for 10-15 minutes

Note: If you need to adjust the intensity of the HIIT then do so. You can alter the run-walk ratios (i.e. run for 30 seconds and walk for 1.5 minutes), or you can decrease the intensity of each run (i.e. run at 6 mph instead of 7.5). And if what I prescribed is too easy, then ramp up the intensity accordingly.

Yes, the fasting keto diet alone will be enough to help you start losing weight; exercise isn't mandatory for it to work. However, exercise will provide you with many additional health benefits, and it'll help you lose more weight (26).

Chapter 10: 42 Keto Friendly Recipes

Bacon Cheeseburger Pie

Ingredients:

- 1lb ground beef
- 2 tsp. onion powder
- 1 tbsp. dry minced onion
- 2 whole eggs
- 1/2 cup mayo
- 1/4 cup heavy cream
- 8 oz. shredded cheddar cheese
- 4 slices bacon

Directions:

1. Brown ground beef on medium low with 1tsp onion powder and 1tbsp minced onion.
2. Drain the fat, season with salt & pepper.
3. Place meat in greased 10" pie plate.
4. Cook bacon to taste then mince into dime-sized portions.
5. Stir 4 oz. shredded cheese with bacon and ground beef.
6. Top with 4 oz. shredded cheese.
7. Whisk mayo, eggs and cream with a dash of pepper.
8. Pour evenly over meat.
9. Bake at 350 degrees F for 30-35 minutes.
10. Let stand for 10 minutes before serving.

Number of servings: 4

Macros (per serving):

Calories: 891.4
Protein: 49.7 g
Carbs: 4.3 g
Fat: 76.7 g

Broiled Tilapia Parmesan

Ingredients:

- 2 thawed tilapia fillets (5 oz. to 6 oz. each)
- 2 tsp. light mayonnaise
- 2 tsp. non-fat plain yogurt
- 1/4 cup shredded parmesan cheese
- 2 to 4 sprigs of fresh dill
- 1 tsp. garlic powder or garlic salt, divided
- Black pepper to taste
- Non-stick cooking spray

Directions:

1. Place mayonnaise, yogurt and parmesan cheese in a small bowl, mix with a spoon until well mixed.
2. Cover a cookie sheet with aluminum and spray with non-stick cooking spray.
3. Set oven to broil on high.
4. Place tilapia fillets onto cookie sheet, about 2 inches apart.
5. Divide the cheese mixture and spread half onto each fillet with a spoon, using the back of the spoon to distribute evenly over fish.
6. Rub dill between your fingers to separate and sprinkle 1 to 2 sprigs worth of leaves over each fillet.
7. Sprinkle each fillet with half of the garlic powder or garlic salt and desired amount of Black Pepper.
8. Place cookie sheet into oven about 6" below the broiler.
9. Watch fish carefully. Depending on the weight of the fillets it will take between 5-7 minutes to cook fully. When the cheese starts to brown, check fish every 30 seconds to see if it's done. Fish will flake easily with a fork when fully cooked.
10. Turn broiler off and leave fish in oven about 5 minutes.

11. Remove from oven and serve with side dishes of your choice.

Number of servings: 2

Macros (per serving):

Calories: 275.2
Protein: 48.5 g
Carbs: 1.4 g
Fat: 8.5 g

Low Carb Cheesecake

Ingredients:

- 2 eggs
- 2 tsp. vanilla extract
- 1 1/2 cups sour cream
- 1/2 cup Splenda granules
- 16 oz. cream cheese, softened
- 2 tbsp. melted butter

Directions:

1. In a large bowl, blend together eggs, vanilla, sour cream and splenda.
2. Slowly add butter and cream cheese.
3. Spoon about 1/2c mix into another bowl and add raspberry flavoring any flavor, sugar free, and mix it well.
4. Spoon remaining mix into a 10 inch spring release pan or 12 ramekins.
5. Add dollops of raspberry batter on top and swirl together thoroughly
6. Bake in 350 degree oven for 20-25 min if cooking ramekins, 35-40 min for spring pan.
7. Place ramekins in a water bath or place a shallow pan with water in oven below the pan or ramekins.

Number of servings: 12

Macros (per serving):

Calories: 231.8
Protein: 4.9 g
Carbs: 3.4 g
Fat: 22.3 g

Cheese and Ham-Stuffed Chicken Breast

Ingredients:

- 4 boneless skinless chicken breasts (4 oz. each)
- 4 slices low sodium ham (1 oz. each)
- 4 slices Fat Free Mozzarella cheese (1 oz. each)
- 1 cup of chopped baby spinach leaves
- 4 tbsp. all purpose flour
- 1 tbsp. extra virgin olive oil
- 1 tbsp. butter
- 1 cup fat free chicken broth
- 1 tbsp. Half-n-Half
- Salt & Pepper to taste

Directions:

1. Preheat oven to 350 F.
2. Cut each breast horizontally almost to the opposite edge. Fold back top half of breast. Sprinkle lightly with salt & pepper. Place 1 slice of ham, 1 slice of mozzarella, & 1/4 cup spinach on each check breast. Fold top half of breasts over filling.
3. Spread 3 tablespoons flour on a plate. Holding chicken breasts closed, coat in flour & remove excess. Add salt and pepper to chicken.
4. Heat oil & margarine and spread in large skillet over medium heat. Place chicken in skillet & cook for 4 minutes on each side or until browned.
5. Transfer chicken to shallow baking dish. Bake in oven for 10 minutes.
6. Whisk chicken broth and cream into remaining 1 TBSP flour in a small bowl. Pour broth mixture into the skillet you browned the chicken in. Heat over medium heat, stirring constantly, until sauce thickens for around 3 minutes
7. Transfer chicken breast to 4 plates and spoon the sauce over the top.

Number of servings: 4

Macros (per serving):

Calories: 271.4
Protein: 39.6 g
Carbs: 5.9 g
Fat: 8.7 g

Ranch Baked Chicken

Ingredients:

- 6 Chicken Breast Bone-in
- 1 cup ranch dressing
- 2 tsp. McCormick's Season salt
- 1 tsp. basil leaves
- 1 tsp. Pepper

Directions:

1. Preheat oven 425 degrees.
2. Rinse chicken breast and place rinsed chicken breast in a 9x13 baking dish
3. Season chicken breast with season salt, pepper, and basil, then pour the dressing over the chicken breast.
4. Cover the baking dish with aluminum foil.
5. Bake 45mins serve and enjoy!

Number of servings: 6

Macros (per serving):

Calories: 191.2
Protein: 9.5 g
Carbs: 1.3 g
Fat: 16.1 g

Egg Muffins

Ingredients:

- 15 large eggs
- 1 green bell pepper
- 1 cup shredded cheddar cheese
- 1/4 cup feta cheese
- Garlic Seasoning to taste

Directions:

1. Preheat oven to 375 F.
2. Spray a silicone pan with non-stick spray. If using a regular muffin pan, use 2 liners.
3. In a bowl, beat the eggs.
4. Add diced veggies and cheese, and then add garlic seasoning to taste.
5. Pour into muffin tins filling 2/3 full.
6. Bake 25-35 minutes until muffins have risen and are slightly browned and set.

Number of servings: 12

Macros (per serving):

Calories: 139.3
Protein: 10.8 g
Carbs: 1.5 g
Fat: 9.8 g

Cheesecake Pancakes

Ingredients:

- 2 large eggs
- 4 oz Cream Cheese
- Splenda to taste
- 1/2 tsp. Cinnamon, ground
- 1 tbsp. flax seed meal

Directions:

1. Place the egg whites in a separate bowl and beat with electric mixer until stiff peaks appear.
2. In a large bowl, put in the cream cheese and beat with the mixer until smooth. Beat in the egg yolks and the sweetener, cinnamon, salt and flaxseed meal.
3. Add in the egg whites.
4. Heat large heavy fry pan over medium low heat, and grease it lightly with butter. Form pancakes using about 1/4 cup of the batter for each pancake. Cook until golden brown on each side.

Number of servings: 2

Macros (per serving):

Calories: 293.5
Protein: 11.1 g
Carbs: 2.1 g
Fat: 26.4 g

Creamy Caesar Mushroom Chicken

Ingredients:

- 3 lbs. of chicken breast, boneless, skinless, and raw, cut in large chunks
- 2 cups of sliced mushrooms
- 8 oz. of creamy caesar dressing
- 4 ounces of low-fat cream cheese
- 11 oz. of cream of chicken soup
- 8 oz. shredded part skim mozzarella cheese

Directions:

1. Pour the bottle of Caesar dressing into the crock pot.
2. Add in the chicken breast chunks and mushrooms to the pot, stir to coat, and cover.
3. Cook on high for about 4 1/2 hours.
4. In a bowl, mix together cream of chicken soup and softened cream cheese.
5. Stir the soup and cream cheese mixture into chicken in crock pot gently.
6. Add mozzarella cheese, and stir it gently.
7. Cook another 1/2 hour until cheese is melted and mixture is hot.
8. Serve and enjoy!

Number of servings: 8

Macros (per serving):

Calories: 493.6
Protein: 50.0 g
Carbs: 4.5 g
Fat: 30.2 g

Grilled Pork Chops

Ingredients:

- 4 boneless and cut pork chops
- 1 tbsp. lite soy sauce
- 2 tsp. minced garlic
- 1/2 tsp. paprika
- 1/2 tsp. salt
- 1/4 tsp. pepper

Directions:

1. Sprinkle pork chops with soy sauce, garlic, paprika, salt and pepper.
2. Cover the pork chops and refrigerate at least 20 minutes or up to 2 hours.
3. Spray grill rack or broiler pan with cooking spray.
4. Preheat grill or broiler.
5. Cook chops 4" from heat, turning once halfway through cooking for 10-12 minutes, or until juices run clear.

Number of servings: 4

Macros (per serving):

Calories: 178.0
Protein: 25.1 g
Carbs: 0.9 g
Fat: 7.4 g

Cranberry Muffins

Ingredients:

- 1-cup whole fresh cranberries
- 1.25-cup flaxseed meal
- 1 tsp. baking powder
- 3 tbsp. cinnamon
- 1 tsp. nutmeg
- 1/2 tsp. salt
- 1/2-cup splenda
- 4 large eggs
- 1/4 cup olive oil
- 1/2 cup Da Vinci's Vanilla sugar free syrup
- 1 tbsp. vanilla

Directions:

1. Preheat oven to 350
2. Generously butter the muffin tins.
3. Pour boiling water over cranberries and let sit for 5 minutes.
4. Mix wet ingredients and dry ingredients separately and then combine them, minus the cranberries.
5. Let the mixture stand for roughly 10 minutes to thicken.
6. Add in cranberries once thickened a tiny bit.
7. Fill each muffin cup up about 1/2-3/4 full.
8. Bake for about 17 minutes or until toothpick comes out clean.

Number of servings: 15

Macros (per serving):

Calories: 110.7
Protein: 4.0 g
Carbs: 5.7 g
Fat: 8.2 g

Crustless Spinach Quiche

Ingredients:

- 1/2 to 1 cup of diced onion
- 1 - 16 oz. package of thawed frozen spinach
- Garlic to taste
- 8 large eggs
- 1/2 cup 2 % cottage cheese
- 2 cups cheddar cheese
- Salt & Pepper to taste

Directions:

1. Preheat oven to 350 Degrees
2. Sauté' onion & garlic, add thawed spinach and cook until most of the moisture is gone.
3. Blend eggs, cottage cheese, and salt and pepper to taste.
4. Add to spinach mixture along with two cups of cheddar cheese.
5. Mix and pour into 9 X 13 greased pan.
6. Bake for 30 minutes until done around edges and a little moist in the center.
7. Serve and enjoy!

Number of servings: 8

Macros (per serving):

Calories: 216.9
Protein: 16.7 g
Carbs: 4.7 g
Fat: 14.7 g

Wilted Spinach Salad

Ingredients:

- 6 oz. fresh baby spinach
- 3 tbsp. cider vinegar
- 1 tbsp. of Splenda
- 1/4 tsp. pepper
- Small pinch of salt
- 6 slices thick bacon, cut in 1/2" pieces
- 1/2 medium red onion, sliced thin (app. 2 ounces)
- 1 clove of minced garlic
- 4 quartered hard boiled eggs

Directions:

1. Place the spinach in a large bowl.
2. In a small bowl, combine the vinegar, Splenda, pepper and salt; set aside.
3. Fry the bacon until crisp. With a slotted spoon, remove the bacon to a paper towel lined plate.
4. Measure out 3 tablespoons bacon grease and get rid of the rest.
5. Heat the bacon grease and sauté the onion for 3 minutes.
6. Add the garlic and cook 15 seconds.
7. Add the vinegar mixture to the skillet and remove from the heat.
8. Rapidly scrape the brown bits off the bottom with a wooden spoon.
9. Pour the hot dressing over the spinach; add the bacon. Toss gently until spinach is slightly wilted.

Number of servings: 4

Macros (per serving):

Calories: 317.7
Protein: 26.1 g

Carbs: 5.4 g
Fat: 21.1 g

Stuffed Jalapeno Peppers

Ingredients:

- 12 medium fresh jalapeno peppers
- 4 oz. of softened cream cheese
- 1, 1/2 cup (6 oz.) finely shredded Cheddar
- 2-3 slices of cooked and thinly chopped bacon
- Jalapeno pepper sauce

Directions:

1. Cut peppers in half lengthwise and remove seeds.
2. Cook peppers in boiling water 5 to 10 minutes and drain well.
3. Combine cheeses with bacon; stack into pepper halves and sprinkle with a couple drops of jalapeno pepper sauce.
4. Place on baking sheet and bake in 400 degrees F oven for 5 minutes until cheese melts.

Number of servings: 4

Macros (per serving):

Calories: 317.7
Protein: 8.5 g
Carbs: 1.8 g
Fat: 12.0 g

Low Carb Deep Dish Pizza

Ingredients:

- 4 oz. softened cream cheese
- 4 eggs
- 1/3 cup heavy cream
- 1/4 cup of grated parmesan cheese
- 1 tbsp. chives
- 1/2 tsp. of pizza seasoning
- 2 cups of shredded cheddar cheese
- 1/2 tsp. garlic
- 1/2 cup of low-carb pizza sauce
- 1-cup mozzarella cheese
- Desired toppings to taste

Directions:

1. Beat together cream cheese and eggs till smooth.
2. Add cream, Parmesan cheese and spices.
3. Spray 13x9" glass baking dish with oil.
4. Place 2 cups of shredded cheese in dish and pour egg mix over.
5. Bake at 375 degrees F for 30 minutes.
6. Spread with sauce and then add your toppings.
7. Cover with mozzarella cheese.
8. Bake till browning and bubbly.
9. Let stand for 5 minutes and enjoy!

Number of servings: 9

Macros (per serving):

Calories: 288.3
Protein: 15.4 g
Carbs: 2.9 g
Fat: 23.6 g

Deviled Eggs

Ingredients:

- 6 large hard boiled eggs
- 2 tbsp. mayonnaise
- 1 tsp. of brown mustard
- Salt and Pepper to taste
- Paprika to taste
- 1 tsp. of finely chopped sweet pickles

Directions:

1. Peel hard-boiled eggs & halve them.
2. Empty hard yolks into a bowl & arrange empty egg whites on a serving dish.
3. Blend egg yolks with all other ingredients and stir until smooth.
4. Fill egg white halves with mixture & sprinkle with paprika for added color.
5. Enjoy!

Number of servings: 6

Macros (per serving):

Calories: 113.4
Protein: 6.3 g
Carbs: 1.0 g
Fat: 9.0 g

Crab Cake Burgers

Ingredients:

- 1 pound crabmeat
- 1 lightly beaten egg
- 1/2 cup panko breadcrumbs
- 1/4 cup light mayonnaise
- 2 tbsp. minced chives
- 1 tbsp. Dijon mustard
- 1 tbsp. lemon juice
- 1 tsp. celery seed
- 1 tsp. onion powder
- 1/4 tsp. freshly ground pepper
- Hot sauce to taste
- 1 tbsp. extra-virgin olive oil
- 2 tsp. of butter

Directions:

1. Blend crab, egg, breadcrumbs, mayonnaise, chives, mustard, lemon juice, celery seed, onion powder, pepper and hot sauce in a large bowl.
2. Form mixture into 6 patties.
3. Heat oil and butter in a large nonstick skillet over medium heat until the butter stops foaming.
4. Cook the patties until golden brown, which will be about 4 minutes per side.

Number of servings: 6

Macros (per serving):

Calories: 159.6
Protein: 11.3 g
Carbs: 5.1 g
Fat: 10.4 g

Lemon Garlic Salmon

Ingredients:

- 2 tbsp. of butter
- 2 tsp. of minced garlic
- 1 tsp. lemon pepper
- 2 (4 oz. each) salmon fillets
- 1 lemon

Directions:

1. Sprinkle salmon fillets on both sides with lemon pepper.
2. In a large skillet, melt butter over medium high heat.
3. Add in garlic.
4. Put salmon in the pan.
5. Cook for 10 minutes per inch of thickness, or until fish flakes when tested with a fork.
6. Flip fillets halfway through cooking to brown other side.
7. Sprinkle with lemon juice before serving.
8. Serve with lemon wedges and a sprig of parsley and enjoy!

Number of servings: 2

Macros (per serving):

Calories: 258.4
Protein: 23.8 g
Carbs: 5.4 g
Fat: 16.7 g

Lemon Rosemary Grilled Chicken Breast

Ingredients:

- 3 tbsp. extra virgin olive oil
- 3 tbsp. of fresh lemon juice
- 3 tbsp. of white wine
- 1 tbsp. of fresh chopped rosemary
- 4 boneless and skinless chicken breasts
- Salt and Pepper to taste

Directions:

1. In a small baking dish, whisk together olive oil, lemon juice, wine and rosemary. Add chicken and turn to coat.
2. Marinate for 45-60 minutes, turning once.
3. Preheat grill and remove chicken breast, season with salt and pepper.
4. Grill chicken over medium high heat until browned, then flip and cook and brown other side.

Number of servings: 4

Macros (per serving):

Calories: 230.2
Protein: 27.3 g
Carbs: 1.2 g
Fat: 11.6 g

Italian Sausage Stuffed Mushrooms

Ingredients:

- App. 40 fresh mushrooms
- 1 lb. of ground Italian sausage
- 8 oz. cream cheese
- 1 can of Rotel
- 1/2 cup mozzarella cheese

Directions:

1. Brown Sausage.
2. Mix in Rotel & Cream Cheese until saucy.
3. Pull out mushroom stems, and scoop out gills.
4. Put mixture into mushrooms & top with mozzarella cheese.
5. Bake at 300 degrees F for 30 minutes.

Number of servings: 10

Macros (per serving):

Calories: 264.3
Protein: 11.0 g
Carbs: 3.2 g
Fat: 23.2 g

Egg Salad

Ingredients:

- 5 large hard boiled eggs
- 2 tbsp. of mayonnaise
- 2 tsp. of Dijon mustard
- Seasonings of choice to taste
- 1/2 tsp. of celery seed
- 1/2 tsp. of black pepper

Directions:

1. Chop eggs
2. Add mayo, mustard and seasonings to taste
3. Serve in Romaine lettuce leaves, atop a mixed green salad, or in a scooped out avocado half and enjoy!

Number of servings: 2

Macros (per serving):

Calories: 292.0
Protein: 15.9 g
Carbs: 1.7 g
Fat: 23.4 g

Blue Cheese Steak

Ingredients:

- 3 tbsp. of crumbled blue cheese
- 1/4 cup of chopped parsley
- 2 tsp. of black, red, and pink cracked peppercorns
- 1, 12 oz. beef fillet, cut into 4, 3 oz. pieces

Directions:

1. Preheat the oven to 375 degrees F.
2. In a small bowl, put the blue cheese and parsley and use a wooden spoon to loosely work into a paste. Cover and refrigerate.
3. Place the cracked peppercorns onto a plate. Pat the meat dry and roll in the peppercorns to coat on all sides.
4. Put a cast-iron skillet or heavy-bottomed ovenproof sauté pan over moderately high heat.
5. Once hot, place steaks into the dry pan and sear the top and bottom of each steak, 1 to 2 minutes per side.
6. Place 1 tablespoon of the blue cheese mixture on top of each steak and transfer the pan to the oven. Roast 6 to 7 minutes for rare, 7 to 8 minutes for medium.

Number of servings: 4

Macros (per serving):

Calories: 245.8
Protein: 18.5 g
Carbs: 1.2 g
Fat: 18.2 g

Fish Nuggets

Ingredients:

- 1/2 cup of finely ground pork rinds
- 1/2 cup of parmesan cheese
- Salt and pepper to taste
- 1 egg
- 1 tbsp. of heavy cream
- 3 frozen vacuum sealed tilapia fillets
- 2 tbsp. of olive oil

Directions:

1. Thaw the fish by letting the still vacuumed fillets sit in a bowl of hot water for a few minutes.
2. Use a food processor or mortar and pestle to finely ground the pork rinds into a powder.
3. In one bowl, thoroughly combine the pork rind powder with the parmesan and whatever spices you like.
4. In a second bowl, whisk the egg and heavy cream.
5. Cut the thawed fish into nuggets (about 1 inch squares.)
6. Heat a skillet to medium-high heat, and then add enough oil to cover the entire surface to a depth of 1/4 inch.
7. Thoroughly cover the fish in the egg mixture on all sides, then thoroughly cover it in the pork rind/cheese mixture and toss it in the oil.
8. Fry until it's golden brown, (about 2-3 minutes) flipping half way through.

Number of servings: 3

Macros (per serving):

Calories: 432.7
Protein: 50.6 g

Carbs: 0.9 g
Fat: 24.3 g

Broccoli Cheddar Soup

Ingredients:

- 2 tsp. of salt
- 3 cups of chicken broth
- 1/2 large chopped onion
- 3 small to medium heads of chopped broccoli
- 1 chopped avocado
- 1 cup of shredded cheddar cheese
- 3 cups of heavy whipping cream

Directions:

1. In a large pot, combine broth, salt, onion, and broccoli, and then bring to a low boil.
2. Lower heat, cover, and simmer for 15 minutes or until the broccoli is nice and soft.
3. Put the ingredients of the pot and the avocado in a big blender of food processor and slightly blend it, or thoroughly puree
4. Return to the pot on medium heat, stir in the cheese and heavy cream, bring it back up to a low boil.
5. Simmer for another 10 minutes or so, stirring regularly and enjoy!

Number of servings: 10

Macros (per serving):

Calories: 347.7
Protein: 5.6 g
Carbs: 7.5 g
Fat: 30.9 g

Cauliflower Crust Pizza

Ingredients:

- 2 cups of raw cauliflower
- 1 cup of shredded mozzarella cheese
- ¼ cup of four cheese alfredo sauce
- 15 pepperoni slices
- 1 large egg
- 1 tsp. of ground Oregano
- 1 tsp. of onion powder
- 1/4 tsp. of garlic salt
- 1 cup of shredded mozzarella cheese

Directions:

1. In a large bowl, grate the raw cauliflower with a cheese grater.
2. Cook in the microwave for about 4 min.
3. Add one cup of shredded mozzarella and stir. Add the egg, onion powder, oregano, and mix with cheese for 30 seconds.
4. On a cookie sheet, place parchment paper to cover sheet and spray non-stick cooking spray generously.
5. Put the dough mixture onto the parchment paper and spread it out toward the edges.
6. Bake for about 15-20 minutes at 450 degrees F.
7. Add your toppings and put back in the oven for about 2-3 min on high broil.

Number of servings: 10

Macros (per serving):

Calories: 274.0
Protein: 17.4 g
Carbs: 5.6 g
Fat: 20.2 g

Peanut Butter Cream Cheese Bites

Ingredients:

- 4 oz. of softened cream cheese
- 1/4 cup of butter
- 2 tbsp. Bell Plantation PB2
- 2 tsp. of swerve

Directions:

1. Mix all ingredients in a bowl.
2. Drop by tablespoon onto parchment paper.
3. Refrigerate for 1 hour and enjoy!

Number of servings: 10

Macros (per serving):

Calories: 84.1
Protein: 1.4 g
Carbs: 1.0 g
Fat: 8.7 g

Almond Bread

Ingredients:

- 3/4 cup almond flour
- 1-1/2 tsp. of baking powder
- 1/4 tsp. of salt
- 1/4 tsp. of garlic powder
- 1/4 tsp. of onion powder
- 5 tsp. of butter
- 2 large eggs.

Directions:

1. Preheat to 375 degrees F.
2. Mix all of the dry ingredients together.
3. Melt the butter in the microwave for 1 minute.
4. Scramble the eggs.
5. Mix the butter and eggs, and add to the dry ingredients.
6. Pour into muffin top pan and bake for 15 minutes.

Number of servings: 8

Macros (per serving):

Calories: 84.1
Protein: 4.3 g
Carbs: 2.6 g
Fat: 6.8 g

Vanilla and Chocolate Fudgesicle

Ingredients:

- 1 scoop of vanilla protein powder
- 4 tsp. coconut oil
- 14 oz. of water
- 14 oz. heavy cream
- 1 scoop of chocolate protein powder
- 8 popsicle molds

Directions:

1. Add vanilla protein powder, 7 oz heavy cream, 7 oz water, and 2 tsp coconut oil to a blender.
2. Blend these items together and place in 4 Popsicle molds.
3. Then add the chocolate protein powder, 7 oz heavy cream, 7 oz water, and 2 tsp coconut oil to the blender and mix together.
4. Pour mixture in remaining 4 Popsicle molds.
5. Refrigerate overnight and enjoy!

Number of servings: 8

Macros (per serving):

Calories: 84.1
Protein: 7.0 g
Carbs: 1.9 g
Fat: 31.4 g

Hot Tuscan Chicken Casserole

Ingredients:

- 2 cups cooked chicken
- 1/4 cooked mashed cauliflower
- 1/2 cup cooked bacon chopped
- 1/3 cup chopped sun dried tomatoes
- 2 tbsp. of lemon juice
- 1/2 tsp. salt
- 1/4 tsp. pepper
- 1 cup of mayonnaise
- 2 tbsp. of red onions
- 1/2 cup of Italian blend cheese

Directions:

1. Preheat oven to 350 degrees F.
2. Cook cauliflower in microwave with 2 tsp water for 10 minutes.
3. Mix all ingredients together minus the chicken, cauliflower and cheese.
4. Add in the chicken and cauliflower to mixture. Spread into a baking dish, and top it off with cheese.
5. Cook for 15 minutes, serve, and enjoy!

Number of servings: 4

Macros (per serving):

Calories: 627.6
Protein: 36.9 g
Carbs: 3.7 g
Fat: 51.5 g

Vanilla Pudding

Ingredients:

- 1 cup heavy cream
- 1 cup whole milk
- 1/4 cup cold water
- 2 tbsp. water
- 2 tbsp. plain gelatin
- 2 tsp. of vanilla extract
- Stevia to taste

Directions:

1. In a sauce pan, heat 2tbsp of water until bubbly.
2. Add milk and heavy cream to the hot pan and heat until very warm.
3. Sprinkle gelatin over 1/4 c water and let sit for 5 minutes.
4. Add softened gelatin to warmed milk and stir until dissolved. Turn off the stove.
5. Stir in vanilla extract and stevia.
6. Pour into serving bowls/cups and chill for about 30-45 minutes until set.

Number of servings: 4

Macros (per serving):

Calories: 255.3
Protein: 4.0 g
Carbs: 4.5 g
Fat: 24.0 g

Fudge

Ingredients:

- 1/4 cup of coconut milk
- 1/2 tsp. of vanilla extract
- 1/2 tsp. salt
- 1/4 cup cocoa powder
- 1 cup of coconut oil
- 5 drops of liquid stevia

Directions:

- Put the coconut oil and coconut milk together in a medium sized bowl and mix with a hand mixer on high for 6 minutes or until well mixed.
- Place the remaining ingredients in the bowl and stir on low speed until the cocoa is added in well. Increase speed and continue mixing until the ingredients are blended together well.
- Place a sheet of parchment or wax paper along the inside of a loaf pan.
- Place the loaf pan in the freezer for at least 15 minutes, until just set.
- Use the edges of the parchment to pull the fudge out of the pan. Place on a cutting board and remove the parchment paper.
- Use a sharp knife to cut the fudge into squares. Store in an airtight container in the freezer.

Number of servings: 12

Macros (per serving):

Calories: 174.8
Protein: 0.4 g
Carbs: 1.3 g
Fat: 19.8 g

Buffalo Chicken Jalapeno Poppers

Ingredients:

- 17 1/2 oz. of chicken thighs
- 4 oz. of bacon
- 2 jalapeno peppers
- 8 oz. of cream cheese
- 8 servings of cheddar cheese
- 16 tsp. of hot sauce
- 6 tbsp. of mayonnaise
- 7 Mason jars

Directions:

1. De-bone all chicken thighs and preheat oven to 400F. Season chicken thighs well with salt and pepper, then lay on a cooling rack over a cookie sheet wrapped in foil. Bake chicken thighs for 40 minutes at 400F.
2. Once the chicken has cooked for 20 minutes, start on the filling. Chop all of the bacon into pieces and put into a pan over medium heat.
3. Once bacon is crispy, add jalapenos into the pan.
4. Once jalapenos are soft and cooked, add cream cheese, mayo, and frank's red hot to the pan. Mix together these ingredients and season to taste.
5. Remove chicken from the oven and let it cool slightly. Once cooled, remove the skins from the chicken.
6. Evenly divide chicken into 7 portions and place in bottom of mason jar.
7. Spread cream cheese mixture over each chicken layer, then top with the sharp Cheddar cheese.
8. Bake for 10-15 minutes at 400 degrees F. Broil for 3-5 minutes to finish.

Number of servings: 7

Macros (per serving):

Calories: 482.9
Protein: 37.0 g
Carbs: 2.7 g
Fat: 53.2 g

Chili

Ingredients:

- 2 tbsp. of chili powder
- 2 tbsp. of cumin seed
- 2 tbsp. of garlic powder
- 16 oz. of fresh, ground pork
- 1 can (6 oz.) of tomato paste
- 16 oz. of lean ground beef
- 2 cups of water
- 8 slices of bacon
- 1 cup of raw red onion
- 1 medium green bell pepper
- 2-1/2 cup of Rotel

Directions:

1. Cut bacon into 1" squares and cook until crisp. Set aside to drain.
2. Chop onion and green pepper and cook in bacon grease until slightly tender. Set aside.
3. Cook ground beef and pork until done.
4. Add cooked onion and pepper, meat, Rotel, tomato paste, and water in Dutch oven.
5. Bring to a boil and cook 15-20 min to meld flavors.
6. Add bacon before serving and enjoy!

Number of servings: 8

Macros (per serving):

Calories: 431.6
Protein: 25.0 g
Carbs: 12.9 g
Fat: 30.5 g

Bacon Cups

Ingredients:

- 12 slices of halved lower-sodium bacon
- 1lb (16 oz.) of lean ground beef
- 4 oz. of cream cheese
- 3/4 cup of shredded colby and monterey jack cheese
- 1/4 tsp. of ground turmeric
- 1/4 tsp. of ground coriander
- 1/4 tsp. of paprika
- 1 tsp. of onion powder
- 2 tsp. of garlic powder
- Salt and Pepper to taste

Directions:

1. Preheat oven to 350 degrees F.
2. Arrange bacon in a lightly greased jumbo muffin pan, with 3-4 pieces per cup.
3. Place the bacon in the oven for approximately 10 minutes or until the edges are crisp
4. Combine the cream cheese and all spices in a bowl until smooth and set to the side.
5. Brown the ground beef in a medium saucepan. When it's almost done, add the cream cheese mixture and simmer until the consistency is the same throughout.
6. Spoon half of the beef mixture into the bacon cups, pressing it firmly into the bottom to hold it tightly.
7. Add half of the shredded cheese on top of the beef.
8. Add the rest of the beef mixture, followed by the rest of the cheese.
9. Bake for an additional 10 minutes or until cheese is golden.
10. Let cool for 5 minutes, serve, and enjoy!

Number of servings: 6

Macros (per serving):

Calories: 391.7
Protein: 22.7 g
Carbs: 2.4 g
Fat: 32.6 g

Lasagna

Ingredients:

- 3 slices of hardwood smoked bacon
- 1 cup of sliced zucchini
- 2 medium red peppers
- 1 oz. cheddar cheese
- 1 oz. monterey cheese
- 2 tomatoes

Directions:

1. Preheat oven to 425 degrees F
2. Slice Zucchini and layer the bottom of glass pan
3. Slice Roma tomatoes and layer over the Zucchini
4. Layer Slices Monterey Cheese over tomatoes
5. Cut Bacon in half and layer along pan
6. Slice Peppers lengthwise and place over bacon
7. Cover with shredded cheddar cheese
8. Cover loosely with tin foil
9. Bake 45 minutes
10. Remove tinfoil and broil for 15 minutes
11. Remove from oven and let stand 10 minutes
12. Serve and enjoy!

Number of servings: 6

Macros (per serving):

Calories: 270.3
Protein: 15.0 g
Carbs: 10.2 g
Fat: 19.4 g

Gnocchi

Ingredients:

- 5 oz. of skim milk mozzarella cheese
- 2 tsp. of parmesan cheese
- 2 large egg yolks

Directions:

1. Melt Parmesan and mozzarella cheese in microwave and mix with any seasonings.
2. Add in egg yolks and mix completely
3. Put in fridge for 10 minutes.
4. Bring a pot of water to a boil.
5. Remove dough from fridge and place on parchment paper, and divide dough into 3 pieces.
6. Roll out each dough ball into a strand around 12 inches long and shape it like a long, fat cylinder.
7. Cut into 1-inch pieces and place in boiling water.
8. When they rise to the top, fry them in a pan to make the edges crispy.
9. Serve and enjoy!

Number of servings: 2

Macros (per serving):

Calories: 255.5
Protein: 21.9 g
Carbs: 2.7 g
Fat: 17.2 g

Cauliflower Casserole

Ingredients:

- 1 med. head of raw (5-6" dia) cauliflower
- 4 oz. cream cheese
- 4 tbsp. of shredded parmesan cheese
- 1/2 cup of sour cream
- 3 slices of hardwood smoked bacon
- 1 stalk of green onion
- 1 cup of shredded cheddar cheese
- 1 tsp. of garlic powder

Directions:

1. Preheat oven to 350 degrees F.
2. Cut cauliflower in small prices and fry bacon.
3. Boil cauliflower to soften it.
4. Mix cream cheese, Parmesan cheese, sour cream, bacon, onions, and garlic powder together.
5. When cauliflower is drained, place on top of cream cheese mixture, and mash it like you would potatoes.
6. Put in 8x8 baking dish. Put cheddar on top and 2 slices of crushed bacon.
7. Cook in oven for 20 minutes.
8. Serve and enjoy!

Number of servings: 9

Macros (per serving):

Calories: 181.8
Protein: 8.0 g
Carbs: 5.3 g
Fat: 14.9 g

Tuna Salad

Ingredients:

- 2 (5-oz.) cans of tuna
- 2/3-cup of minced celery
- 2 tbsp. of minced sweet onion
- 1-1/2 tbsp. of diced pimiento
- 1/4-cup dill pickle relish
- 1/2-cup of mayonnaise
- 3/4 of a small, ripe avocado
- 2 hard-boiled and finely chopped eggs

Directions:

1. Mash ripe avocado and mayonnaise together.
2. Place all ingredients in large bowl and blend thoroughly.
3. Chill before serving and enjoy!

Number of servings: 4

Macros (per serving):

Calories: 338.4
Protein: 17.3 g
Carbs: 5.5 g
Fat: 26.7 g

Swiss Chicken Bake

Ingredients:

- 1 oz. of swiss cheese
- 16 oz. of boneless and skinless chicken breast
- 8 tbsp. of mayonnaise
- 8 tbsp. of sour cream
- 12 tbsp. grated parmesan cheese

Directions:

1. Preheat oven to 375 degrees F.
2. Pat chicken dry and put in a greased 9x13 pan.
3. Add sliced cheese on top of chicken breasts.
4. In a bowl blend together mayonnaise, sour cream, 2/3 of the Parmesan cheese, salt, pepper and garlic powder.
5. Spread this over chicken and add remaining Parmesan cheese on top.
6. Bake for 40-50 minutes.
7. Serve and enjoy!

Number of servings: 4

Macros (per serving):

Calories: 576.6
Protein: 43.1 g
Carbs: 2.0 g
Fat: 43.5 g

Kale Frittata

Ingredients:

- 3 tsp. of bacon grease
- 1 cup of zucchini
- 3 cups of raw kale
- 1 cup of spinach
- 3 oz. black forest ham
- 8 large eggs
- 2 oz. Romano cheese

Directions:

1. Preheat oven to 370 degrees F.
2. Sauté chopped vegetables in bacon grease.
3. Add in the ham and cheese.
4. Lightly beat the eggs and add them in the mixture.
5. Cook on low heat until the bottom is set, which will be about 4-5 minutes.
6. Bake for 25 - 30 minutes, serve, and enjoy!

Number of servings: 4

Macros (per serving):

Calories: 284.1
Protein: 23.0 g
Carbs: 9.1 g
Fat: 17.4 g

Taco Soup

Ingredients:

- 8 oz. of cream cheese
- 1/2 cup of heavy whipping cream
- 1 tsp. of chili powder
- 1 lb. of raw ground turkey
- 1 can of chicken broth
- 2 garlic cloves
- 1 large, raw onion
- 2 medium (app. 3/5" diameter) tomatoes
- 1 tbsp. cumin

Directions:

1. Brown the pound of ground turkey.
2. Drain the meat and add in two minced garlic cloves and half a cup of onions.
3. Stir those in and then add in one tablespoon of cumin and one teaspoon of chili powder.
4. While the spices soak, dice up an eight-ounce block of cream cheese and your tomatoes.
5. Add in the cream cheese and use the back of a wooden spoon to mash it into the meat.
6. When the cream cheese completely coats the meat, add in tomatoes, chicken broth and half a cup of heavy cream. Stir the mixture well and bring ingredients to a boil.
7. Serve and enjoy!

Number of servings: 8

Macros (per serving):

Calories: 359.4
Protein: 25.7 g
Carbs: 5.2 g
Fat: 26.4 g

Bacon Cheddar Meatloaf

Ingredients:

- 32 oz. 80/20 ground beef chuck
- 1 tbsp. dried minced onions
- 1 tsp. of garlic powder
- 1 tsp. of minced garlic
- 1 tsp. of mustard
- 8 tbsp. of BBQ Sauce
- 1 large raw egg
- 1-1/2 cup shredded fiesta blend cheese
- 5 servings of your choice of turkey bacon

Directions:

1. Preheat oven to 400 degrees F.
2. Combine all the ingredients for the meat and press into the bottom of a greased 9 x 13 casserole dish.
3. Brush the barbecue sauce on top and sprinkle the cheese and bacon on top.
4. Bake for 30-40 minutes.
5. Serve and enjoy!

Number of servings: 8

Macros (per serving):

Calories: 368.9
Protein: 25.6 g
Carbs: 2.9 g
Fat: 27.8 g

Coconut Shrimp

Ingredients:

- 1/2 cup of coconut milk
- 1/2 cup of heavy whipping cream
- 1 cup of unsweetened coconut flakes
- 16 oz. of cooked shrimp
- 1 tsp. of almond extract
- 1 tsp. of apple cider vinegar
- 1 tsp. of coconut extract
- 1/2 tsp. of vanilla extract
- 1 tbsp. of Splenda
- 3 cups of cooked broccoli florets
- 1 tbsp. of olive oil

Directions:

1. Add olive oil to pan over med to high heat.
2. Add shrimp and cook 2-3 minutes, add almond extract and apple cider vinegar, cook 1 more minute.
3. Remove shrimp from pan.
4. Add coconut milk, heavy cream, and Swerve. Cook for about 5 minutes until reduced by half.
5. Add back shrimp and add coconut extract and vanilla extract. Then cook for an additional 1-2 minutes.
6. Remove from heat. Add in cooked broccoli.
7. Top with unsweetened coconut flakes.
8. Serve and enjoy!

Number of servings: 8

Macros (per serving):

Calories: 274.5
Protein: 14.5 g
Carbs: 9.0 g
Fat: 20.0 g

Chapter 11: Frequently Asked Questions

Do I have to do both the fasting diet and the keto diet at the same time?

No, you certainly don't have to combine the diets and do them both at the same time if you don't want to. You can still get great results from doing only intermittent fasting or the ketogenic diet by itself. The main thing you need to focus on is burning off more calories than you consume. If only following one of the two diets at a time makes things easier for you to follow through, then by all means do it.

How much weight should I lift during the workouts?

Lift as much weight as you possibly can for the given rep range. Initially, you won't know how much weight to use so you'll have to take your best guess. For example, let's say you're doing bench press for 8 reps. You think you can lift around 150 pounds for that many reps, but on your first set you easily complete 10 reps.

This means the weight is too light and you need to increase it for the next set. On the next set you lift 165 pounds and struggle to complete the 8th rep. This is what you want to happen and it means you've found a good weight to use. Once you can complete all 3 sets for 8 reps with 165 pounds, move up to 170 the next time you bench press. If you can't complete 8 reps for all 3 sets stick with 165 until you can. Here's an example:

Workout 1: Bench Press with 165 pounds
Set 1: 8 reps
Set 2: 8 reps
Set 3: 7 reps

Because you only completed 7 reps on the last set, stick with 165 for the next workout—

Workout 2: Bench Press with 165 pounds
Set 1: 8 reps
Set 2: 8 reps
Set 3: 8 reps

Because you completed all 3 sets for 8 reps move up to 170 on your next workout with bench press.

Note: It's better to use a weight that's too heavy and miss a rep or two than it is to use a weight that's too light and leave some reps in the tank. For example, it's better to do 170 pounds and only complete 6 reps instead of 8 opposed to using 155 pounds and stopping at 8 reps even though you could've easily done more reps.

How Fast Should I Lose Weight?

The more weight you have to lose, the faster the rate at which you can lose the weight. For example, if you have 50+ pounds to lose, you can lose weight at a rate of 2 pounds or more per week. If you only have 5 pounds to lose, then you'll lose weight at a rate of .5 pound per week.

For most people, losing 1 pound per week is the sweet spot. You'll be creating an average caloric deficit of 500 calories daily. At this pace, you'll be losing weight fairly quickly and you won't be miserable all of the time from a complete lack of calories.

What Am I Allowed to Drink During a Fast?

The only drinks you're allowed to have during a fast are drinks that contain zero to a few calories (10 or less). Drinking something like a soda or orange juice would break the fast and stop all of the benefits from the fast. Here's a list of acceptable drinks you can have during a fast:

- Water
- Green Tea
- Black Coffee
- Diet Soda
- Water Flavorings that Don't Contain any Calories

What Should I Eat When I'm Not Fasting?

This is a tricky question to answer, and it relates to that old phrase, "If you give a man a fish, you feed him for a day, but if you teach him how to fish you feed him for life." If I tell you what to eat for every meal, than I am giving you a fish.

You're not going to learn anything. You won't know how to adapt and eat if you're away from home for example. But if I teach you *how* to eat, then I can teach you how to stay lean for the rest of your life. I'll give you some guidelines to follow, but don't feel the need to stick with them 100% of the time:

Guideline #1: Above all else—burn off more calories than you consume.

Nothing else matters if you're not in a caloric deficit. Many people seem to forget about this and think if they eat healthy, then they're guaranteed to lose weight. Yes, healthy foods are *generally* lower in calories than unhealthy foods, but eating healthy doesn't guarantee anything. Being in a caloric deficit will guarantee weight loss.

Guideline #2: Forgive yourself

Understand there will be times when you slip up and that's ok. What's not ok is to make the situation worse by saying, "screw it," and binge eating everything in sight. Give yourself permission to be human and make mistakes. Don't strive to be perfect 100% of the time, aim for 85%, and even when you don't reach 85%, forgive yourself.

Back when I was 16 and I first started working out, I would feel incredibly guilty if I even thought about eating a cookie. I would take pride in myself because I could resist temptation while others couldn't. But fitness felt like a chore, and I wasn't having fun with it. Don't be perfect—be the human that you are!

Guideline #3: Fill up on the healthy stuff first

Sometimes I'll be hungry for ice cream, but I'll tell myself I can only eat after I finish the rest of my meal. At times, I won't even end up eating any ice cream because I wasn't hungry for it after the main course. There will be times when you'll crave certain foods, but filling up on your main course first can help to stop those cravings.

Foods high in protein like chicken breast and steak work great for this. These foods require a lot of chewing before you can swallow them, which will slow you down. High protein foods are also very satiating, so you might get full before you satisfy your sweet tooth.

Guideline #4: Know yourself and spread out your calories accordingly

Let's say you determine you need to eat 1,800 calories daily to lose weight. You'll do intermittent fasting for the first part of the day, and then eat 3 meals usually around 1:00, 5:00, and 9:00. You could bust up your allotted calories evenly, and eat 600 calories for each of your 3 meals, but you certainly don't have to.

For example, let's say you like to eat bigger meals later in the day before you go to bed. You could eat less calories during your first 2 meals and save the extra calories for your last meal when you would actually want to eat them. For instance:

Meal 1: 400 calories
Meal 2: 400 calories
Meal 3: 1,000 calories

Change this up based on however it is you like to eat. If you like eating more of your calories earlier in the day, then do so, but eat less at night. You don't have to evenly distribute your calories across meals if you don't want to.

Is there anything in particular I should eat to break my fast with?

No. Once you've completed your fast for the day, eat whatever meal you'd normally eat that follows your ketogenic diet plan. It's kind of like coming back from the dentist after a teeth cleaning. You don't want to ruin that sparkly clean feeling, but something has to end it. Fasting is no different.

How much water should I drink on a daily basis?

Your body is made up of about 60% water, so it's important to consume water for several reasons:

- It'll help keep your joints and ligaments fluid, which can help prevent injury.
- Water can help control your caloric intake.
- Flush out toxins
- Improve skin quality
- Improve kidney function
- Improve your focus

Many people recommend that you should drink 1 gallon of water per day. This is a blanket answer that doesn't meet individual needs. This recommendation would have a 100-pound woman drinking the same amount of water as a 200-pound man. Absurd!

Other health experts advise drinking eight 8-ounce glasses (64 ounces total) of water a day. But again 64 ounces isn't going to be enough for most people. What should you do then? I don't keep track of my water intake—I go by how I feel and the color of my urine.

Your body's own thirst mechanism will be accurate in telling you if you need more water. If you feel thirsty, then go drink some water. If not, then you're probably ok. You can also use the color of your urine to judge how hydrated you are. If your urine is yellow, then you should drink more water. If it's clear, then you should be good to go. This keeps things simple and it's one less thing you have to keep track of.

How Do I Motivate Myself to Go to the Gym?

Finding the motivation to go to the gym or eat right can be hard. No matter who you are, there will be times when you don't feel like working out. Having that feeling is ok, but you can't let it control you. There will be times when you'll have to do it anyway, even when you don't feel like it.

That's what will ultimately separate a long-term successful fitness journey from failing at it. I do have some tips to help you out along the way however:

Tip #1: Focus on Gradual Improvements

Many people make fitness an all-or-nothing game. They tell themselves that they'll workout 5 days a week and eat clean 100% of the time for the rest of their lives. Let's say you workout only 4 days one week. Are you a failure?

Of course not. You still worked out 4 days, but in your mind you are because you failed to reach 5 workouts. You make it hard to celebrate any small successes that you do have because the standards are too high.

Instead, focus on making smaller, more gradual improvements, and celebrate any successes you have along the way. For example, start off with a goal to only workout 2 days per week if it's been years since you've last worked out. Once you achieve that goal, you'll feel good about yourself, and you can move up to working out 3 days per week and so on.

Tip #2: Action Leads Motivation

People think they have to get the inspiration or motivation from somewhere in order to take the action necessary to workout. The reverse of that is actually true. You need to start by taking an action no matter how small. And once you get started, you'll likely want to continue on with what you're doing.

When I think about everything I have to do to workout: put my gym clothes on, drive to the gym, workout with a bunch of grueling exercises, drive back, and shower—I start to make up silly excuses as to why I should skip this time. Instead, I'll tell myself to do just one exercise when I get to the gym and not pressure myself to do anything more. After I finish that first exercise, it's always easier for me to finish the rest of the workout.

You just have to get started. Try this out for any healthy habit you want to start. For example, if you want to start flossing your teeth, tell yourself you'll only floss one tooth and don't pressure yourself to do anything more than that!

Tip #3: Put Your Own Money on the Line

Money is a very powerful motivator. And you can use your own money to motivate yourself to start working out more. Here's what you're going to do—give someone a good amount of money. Not $20, but something that would actually hurt you—$100, $200, $500, or whatever you can't afford to lose.

Then tell your friend that if you don't go to the gym 3 days this week, they get to keep the money. When you give up the money in the first place, you'll fight to get it back. This is much different than telling yourself you'll give the money to someone after you miss your workouts.

It's too easy to make an excuse and not give away the money. Give the money up in the first place and make sure your friend actually holds you accountable to it. This is by far the best way to get motivation to workout. There's a real cost involved if you don't comply. You'll either get ripped or go broke trying.

Conclusion

Thanks for reading this book all the way to the end! I firmly believe that it's truly possible for you to achieve a healthy and good-looking body that you're proud of by following the nutritional and training advice outlined in this book. Getting fit isn't easy, but it's worth it. Stay strong and persist even when you mess up, and you'll succeed in the long run.

Finally, if you have any questions please be sure to email me at thomas@rohmerfitness.com. I'd be more than happy to answer any questions that you have!

Sources

(1)http://fitness.mercola.com/sites/fitness/archive/2016/03/25/health-benefits-fasting.aspx#_edn1

(2) https://www.ncbi.nlm.nih.gov/pubmed/371355

(3)https://www.ncbi.nlm.nih.gov/pmc/articles/PMC3289210/

(4)https://www.ncbi.nlm.nih.gov/pmc/articles/PMC329619/

(5)https://www.ncbi.nlm.nih.gov/pmc/articles/PMC4257368/

(6)https://www.ncbi.nlm.nih.gov/pubmed/24993615

(7)https://www.ncbi.nlm.nih.gov/pubmed/17929537

(8)https://www.ncbi.nlm.nih.gov/pmc/articles/PMC1204764/

(9)https://www.ncbi.nlm.nih.gov/pubmed/8116550

(10)
https://www.ncbi.nlm.nih.gov/pubmed/15148063

(11)
https://www.ncbi.nlm.nih.gov/pmc/articles/PMC4125607/

(12)
https://www.ncbi.nlm.nih.gov/pmc/articles/PMC333231/

(13)
https://www.ncbi.nlm.nih.gov/pubmed/15767618

(14)
https://www.ncbi.nlm.nih.gov/pubmed/22905670

(15)
https://www.ncbi.nlm.nih.gov/pubmed/17313687

(16)
http://ajcn.nutrition.org/content/77/5/1146.short

(17)
https://www.ncbi.nlm.nih.gov/pubmed/16409560

(18)
https://www.ncbi.nlm.nih.gov/pubmed/12088525

(19)
http://ajprenal.physiology.org/content/293/4/F974

(20)
https://www.ncbi.nlm.nih.gov/pubmed/17228046

(21)https://www.ncbi.nlm.nih.gov/pubmed/22825659

(22)
https://www.ncbi.nlm.nih.gov/pubmed/23521346

(23)
https://www.ncbi.nlm.nih.gov/pubmed/22460474

(24)
https://www.ncbi.nlm.nih.gov/pubmed/2796409

(25)
https://www.ncbi.nlm.nih.gov/pubmed/8028502

(26)
https://www.ncbi.nlm.nih.gov/pmc/articles/PMC1402378/

*Recipes courtesy of users at Sparkrecipes.com

32519742R00061

Printed in Great Britain
by Amazon